RAISING A CHILD WITH DIABETES

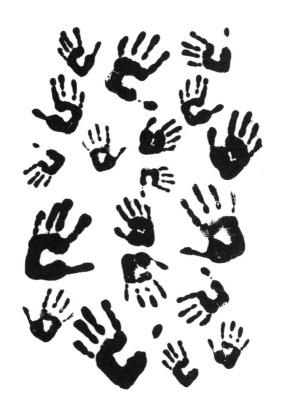

A Guide for Parents

RAISING A CHILD WITH DIABETES

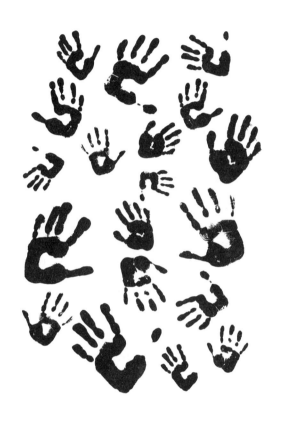

A Guide for Parents

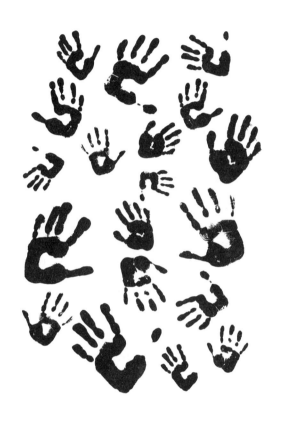 American Diabetes Association.

LINDA SIMINERIO, RN, MS, CDE
JEAN BETSCHART, RN, MN, CDE

Publisher: Susan H. Lau
Editorial Director: Peter Banks
Book Acquisitions Manager: Susan Reynolds
Book Editors: Sherrye Landrum, Karen Ingle
Production Manager: Carolyn R. Segree

Page design and typesetting services by Insight Graphics, Inc.
Cover design by Heidi Fixler Verges.
Writing assistance by Eleanor Mayfield.
Editorial and project management by Christine B. Welch,
Off-Press Publishing.

Printed in the United States of America

American Diabetes Association
1660 Duke Street
Alexandria, VA 22314

Library of Congress Cataloging-in-Publication Data

Siminerio, Linda M.
Raising a child with diabetes : a guide for parents / Linda Siminerio,
Jean Betschart.
p. cm.
Includes bibliographical references and index.
ISBN 0-945448-48-1 (pbk.)
1. Diabetes in children—Popular works. 2. Diabetes in children—
Patients—Home care. I. Betschart, Jean. II. Title.
RJ420.D5S57 1995
618.92'462—dc20   95-17266   CIP

Table of Contents

For most folks, parenthood is a challenge all by itself. Adding the tasks of diabetes care to normal parenting responsibilities makes the job even bigger. You will need help along the way to manage it all.

Help can come in many forms: as friends and relatives who support you; in a strong, caring medical team; and through learning as much as you possibly can about diabetes. This book is intended to help give you support and knowledge so that you will be prepared to handle issues that come up in the daily life of your child with diabetes. It also approaches care issues as they change as your child grows. Use it as a reference book. If your child has a sick day or is being a picky eater, you can reread the parts on how to deal with these issues.

The best diabetes care changes to meet the needs of the individual. It changes as your child grows and develops. Food likes and dislikes come and go. Children pick up different hobbies and sports. Your approach to diabetes care will need to be flexible, based on the needs of your child, the philosophy of your health-care team, and your own parenting style. Therefore, use the guidance here in conjunction with the advice of your health-care providers. There are many approaches to treating diabetes; if you are currently doing something different from what is recommended here, it does not mean that one way is right and the other wrong. The *right* approach is the one that works best for your child. And sometimes the only way of knowing which is best is to try several different approaches.

Two notes: We have alternated the use of he and she by chapters to avoid having to repeat the awkward "he or she" when referring to your child. Also, any mention of a brand name product does not imply endorsement of the product by us or the American Diabetes Association. We use brand names only as examples of the kinds of products available.

We extend special thanks to our families for their constant support of our endeavors to promote diabetes care, to the members of the Children's Hospital of Pittsburgh Diabetes Care Team for their encouragement, and to the American Diabetes Association for their pursuit of excellence.

Linda dedicates this book to the loving memory of her father John A. Mulac.

Linda Siminerio, RN, MS, CDE
Jean Betschart, RN, MN, CDE

When you learn that your child has diabetes, you may feel as if your world has turned upside down. There is so much information to absorb and so many questions that don't have good answers. This book will help you and your family learn about diabetes. Once you've read this book and started attending a diabetes education program, you'll begin to understand why so many people can face life with diabetes positively.

Why does your child have this disease? Was it something you did? Could it have been prevented? What do you do now? Your much-loved child is dependent on insulin injections several times a day to stay alive. He needs blood tests all of the time. What about the rest of your family, your other children? You can't believe your life will ever be normal again.

And you're right. Your life won't ever be the way it was before. In time, however, you'll achieve a different kind of normality—one that includes blood test strips, emergency supplies of orange juice, syringes, and all the other paraphernalia of life with diabetes.

Diabetes can be a very unpredictable disease. You can do everything right, follow all the instructions from your doctor and dietitian, and your child's blood glucose levels may still not be where you want them to be. On the other hand, things may go well when you least expect them to, such as when your child's schedule is off.

As a parent you may feel it's your fault that your child has diabetes. You may think that you could have done something to prevent it. However, even if you had known that your child was genetically at risk for diabetes, there is currently no proven way of preventing the disease from occurring.

Children sometimes feel that getting diabetes is some kind of punishment for bad behavior. It's important to talk to your child to find out how he feels and to help him understand that nothing you or he did *caused* the diabetes.

Diabetes can't be cured—yet. But it *can* be controlled. New and better kinds of insulin are available. Easy-to-use glucose meters make it possible for children to check their own blood glucose levels. New knowledge gained from research tells us that diabetes treatment can be flexible—that rigid diets and schedules are not always necessary.

The good news is that you *can* cope. With knowledge, determination, and good medical care, your child with diabetes can lead a life that is as healthy, active, and fun filled as that of any of his friends. We hope that the information in this book helps you and your child to achieve this goal.

Diabetes mellitus is not a new disorder. It was around as early as 30 A.D. Diabetes is a Greek word that means "to run through." Mellitus is a Latin word that means "honeyed." Healers coined this term to describe what they saw: People with diabetes urinated a lot and their urine was sweet.

We now know that diabetes occurs when the body cannot use and store food properly. Food is broken down during digestion so the body can use it for energy. Proteins become amino acids. Carbohydrates become glucose. Fat becomes fatty acids. These substances enter your bloodstream and travel to where your body needs them.

Glucose is the body's main energy source. Before it can be used as energy, glucose must get inside all of the body's cells. Insulin is the key that opens the "doors" on the cell wall, letting the glucose in.

In people with diabetes, either the body does not make insulin or it cannot use the insulin available. As a result, instead of entering the cells, glucose stays in the blood. The cells starve, and glucose levels in the blood rise. High glucose levels in the blood are a sign that a person has diabetes.

The two most common types of diabetes are **insulin-dependent** (type I) and **non-insulin-dependent** (type II) diabetes. In insulin-dependent (type I) diabetes, the body doesn't make insulin. People with this type of diabetes depend on daily injections of insulin to survive. Most children have type I diabetes, but adults may get it too.

In non-insulin-dependent (type II) diabetes, the body makes insulin but doesn't use it properly. Type II diabetes mostly affects adults; it is extremely rare in children. Many of the signs of high blood glucose are the same in both type I and type II diabetes. People with type II diabetes often can manage their diabetes through diet or by taking a pill to control their blood glucose levels. Sometimes they may also need to take insulin.

In the past, type I diabetes was called **juvenile-onset** and type II was known as **maturity-onset** diabetes. These names were changed because they were misleading. This book is about type I diabetes.

Diabetes is one of the most common chronic diseases in children. Of the estimated 300,000 Americans who have type I diabetes, about 123,000 of these are children younger than age 20. One in every 600 children develops diabetes. Every year about 13,000 new cases of type I diabetes are diagnosed in people under 20 years of age. About 16,000 people 20 years or older get type I diabetes each year.

THE PANCREAS

To understand type I diabetes you need to know about the pancreas, a large gland located behind the stomach.

The pancreas has two main jobs in the body. It makes digestive juices and chemicals called enzymes that help the body to break down food into substances the body can use for fuel. The pancreas also makes hormones that help to deliver fuel to cells. One of these hormones is insulin, which helps to deliver glucose to cells.

Insulin is made by clusters of cells in the pancreas called the **islets of Langerhans**. The islets contain **beta cells**, which make insulin. Type I diabetes occurs when something damages the beta cells, causing the body to gradually stop making insulin. Without insulin, the body cannot use glucose for energy. Insulin injections replace the missing insulin and allow the body to use glucose.

CAUSES OF TYPE I DIABETES

For unknown reasons, the body sometimes rejects and destroys its own cells. This process is called an **autoimmune attack**. When the body attacks and destroys the beta cells, the pancreas can no longer make insulin.

The autoimmune attack may be triggered by a virus. Many children who get diabetes do so shortly after having a viral illness. The peak seasons for the diagnosis of diabetes in children are September (when school begins and children are more exposed to viruses from other children) and January–February (when a lot of viruses are around and many people get viral illnesses).

Scientists don't know exactly how a virus might lead to diabetes. However, they do know that some people inherit a higher risk for type I diabetes. People often wonder why, in some families, more than one person has diabetes. The reason is that, in those families, family members share the genes that make them prone to diabetes.

But genes alone do not seem to cause type I diabetes. It's possible that in people whose genes make them prone to diabetes, a virus somehow flips the switch that "turns on" diabetes. However, a virus alone is almost certainly not enough to cause diabetes. Thousands of children get viral infections every year, and only a few of them get diabetes.

Some people, especially children, worry that they can "catch" diabetes from contact with someone who has it. **Diabetes is not contagious. It cannot be transmitted from one person to another.**

SIGNS AND SYMPTOMS OF DIABETES

The symptoms of diabetes are caused by blood glucose levels that are too high (**hyperglycemia**). If high blood glucose is not treated it may develop into **ketoacidosis**, a very serious condition.

Hyperglycemia (high blood glucose)

Insulin helps to move glucose from the blood into the body's cells. When food is eaten, the body breaks it down into more glucose. Blood glucose levels can get too high when

- ◆ the body gets too little insulin, too much food, or too little exercise
- ◆ the body is under physical stress from a cold, sore throat, or other illness
- ◆ the child is feeling emotional stress (for example, worrying about a test at school)

When your child was diagnosed with diabetes she may have had some or all of the following signs and symptoms, which indicate that her blood glucose level is too high.

- ◆ **Frequent urination.** When your child has diabetes, high glucose in the blood filters into the urine, pulling water with it. This creates a large volume of urine and makes your child urinate a lot.
- ◆ **Excessive thirst.** The body is losing so much water in urine that it becomes dehydrated, causing your child to feel very thirsty.

- **Weight loss.** Your child may lose weight because the body, unable to make proper use of food, tries to get nourishment by burning stored fat for energy. Weight loss may also occur because the body is losing so much water in urine.
- **Increased appetite.** This is the body's way of asking for the food it needs to gain weight and replace calories lost in urine.
- **Tiredness and weakness.** Your child may feel tired and weak because the body's cells are dehydrated and starving. Muscles and other tissues are depleted of glucose and water.
- **Vision problems.** Your child may complain of difficulty seeing the chalkboard or reading signs at a distance. High blood glucose can cause the lens of the eye to change shape, leading to blurred vision. This does not cause permanent eye damage. Once blood glucose is under control, vision will improve.

You will learn to recognize the signs and symptoms of hyperglycemia in your child. For how to prevent and treat hyperglycemia, see page 69.

Ketoacidosis and diabetic coma

Without insulin, glucose cannot enter the body's cells to provide energy. The cells are forced to burn fat to get the energy they need. When fat is burned, by-products called **ketones** build up in the blood and spill into the urine.

Small amounts of ketones are probably not harmful. However, when ketones build up they can poison the body. A high level of ketones in the blood and urine is called **ketoacidosis**. The most common causes of ketoacidosis are:

- undiagnosed or newly diagnosed diabetes
- illness
- too little insulin to meet the body's needs

Ketoacidosis usually does not develop without warning. The signs and symptoms of ketoacidosis are:

- ketones in the urine and blood
- dehydration (symptoms include sunken eyes; dry, cracked lips; dry mouth; skin that remains "pinched up" after it is pinched)
- nausea and vomiting

- ◆ fruity-smelling breath
- ◆ labored or heavy breathing
- ◆ abdominal pain
- ◆ drowsiness

If your child develops any of these symptoms, it's extremely important to contact your doctor right away. If left untreated, ketoacidosis can lead to a coma. However, a person can have ketoacidosis without being in a coma. With prompt treatment, children usually recover completely from ketoacidosis. For more on preventing and treating ketoacidosis, see page 70.

HYPOGLYCEMIA (LOW BLOOD GLUCOSE)

Hypoglycemia (low blood glucose) is common in children with diabetes. It is the exact opposite of hyperglycemia (high blood glucose). Low blood glucose occurs when your child has too much insulin, not enough food (or if food is eaten late), or more exercise than usual.

When blood glucose starts to drop too low, adrenaline (a hormone that helps the body deal with emergencies) jumps into action to try to raise it. When this happens, your child may show the following signs and symptoms, which are related to this rush of adrenaline:

- ◆ shakiness
- ◆ pale, clammy skin
- ◆ hunger
- ◆ sweating
- ◆ rapid pulse

Most of the time hypoglycemia is mild and can be easily treated by giving the child a sweet food. In severe hypoglycemia the brain is deprived of glucose, causing the following symptoms:

- ◆ irritability, crying
- ◆ personality changes
- ◆ poor coordination
- ◆ dizziness
- ◆ fatigue, sleepiness, unconsciousness
- ◆ headache
- ◆ confusion
- ◆ nightmares
- ◆ seizures

Just as you will learn to recognize the symptoms of high blood glucose in your child, you will also learn to recognize the symptoms of low blood glucose. For how to prevent and treat hypoglycemia, see page 65.

KEEPING BLOOD GLUCOSE IN A TARGET RANGE

Years ago, people with diabetes did not have the tools they needed to control their condition well. But now people with diabetes can do things that make diabetes easier to control, like frequently checking their blood glucose levels. Some of the new glucose meters are so easy to use that a young child can learn to do his own tests.

In the past, people with diabetes were advised to stick to a rigid diet. Now, however, we know that diabetes can be successfully managed with a flexible approach that keeps blood glucose levels within a target range by balancing food, insulin, and exercise and testing glucose levels regularly.

What's more, a diet that's healthy for your child with diabetes is healthy for your whole family. That means everyone can eat the same meals.

Science has created new products that make diabetes easier to manage. With artificial sweeteners, children with diabetes can enjoy sweet-tasting foods and drinks without raising their blood glucose levels too high. New kinds of insulin have been developed that are much less likely to cause allergic reactions.

It takes energy and motivation to keep on top of diabetes management, but with education and support you and your child will learn to live successfully with diabetes.

You and your child will have some good days and some frustrating days. Diabetes can be unpredictable. Sometimes things may not go well even when you do everything right. On the other hand, glucose levels may stay in range when you don't expect them to, such as on a day when your child has different foods to eat or her usual schedule is disrupted.

Understanding how diabetes works in your child can help to give you the confidence you need to try to solve problems as they arise.

Having diabetes can affect many aspects of your child's life and your life as a family. Most of the day-to-day care of a child with diabetes is carried out by family members and by the child when he is old enough. Sharing the responsibilities of care among family members can be helpful because that way nobody "burns out."

In caring for your child with diabetes, it's important to take into account your child's personality, likes and dislikes, and so on. No two children with diabetes are alike or treated in exactly the same way. It's also important that caring for your child with diabetes fits into your family's life (as well as your child's school schedule and social life), not the other way around.

Each child with diabetes will have a treatment plan designed for him and his family's schedule. The goal of treatment is to keep your child's blood glucose levels within a target range by balancing insulin with food and exercise. Treatment plans include:

♦ insulin injections
♦ blood glucose testing
♦ meal planning

Treatment also helps to maintain your child's overall good health by paying attention to all of the following:

♦ blood glucose testing and treatment of high and low blood glucose levels when they occur
♦ your child's growth and development
♦ your child's success in school and with friends
♦ the whole family's ability to cope with life with diabetes

NEW THINKING ABOUT TREATING CHILDREN WITH DIABETES

Ideas about how to treat children with diabetes have changed a lot in recent years. Some of the new thinking is the result of a 10-year study called the Diabetes Control and Complications Trial (DCCT).

This study showed that keeping blood glucose levels as close to normal as possible can postpone or prevent complications that are caused by diabetes. Complications occur very rarely in children, but they can affect people who have had diabetes for 15 years or more.

Young children did not take part in the DCCT. The participants were all between the ages of 13 and 39 when they entered the study. Because none of the study volunteers were children, we can't say for sure whether the study's results apply to children.

"Tight glucose control"—trying to keep glucose levels as close to normal as possible all the time—is usually not recommended for very young children, who may have episodes of low blood glucose that are undetected because they cannot tell their parents when they feel "low." In general, however, diabetes health-care professionals agree that achieving an improvement in glucose control is beneficial for everyone with diabetes.

It's reasonable to try to achieve good control in children as long as frequent or severe hypoglycemia does not occur. "Good control" means keeping blood glucose levels within a target range that is considered best for your child.

Your doctor and diabetes educator will work with you to determine your child's target range. A normal blood glucose level is between 70 mg/dl and 120 mg/dl. If your child is a mature, motivated 14-year-old, that range may be a reasonable goal for him. However, in a two-year-old who can't tell you when he feels "low," trying to keeping the glucose level in the normal range may be unrealistic and may actually cause episodes of low blood glucose.

Developing a treatment plan that meets your child's individual needs, including his eating habits, activity level, and schedule, can help to keep blood glucose levels within the target range. Among most children and teenagers who succeed in keeping their glucose levels within a target range most of the time, the following practices are common:

♦ They eat reasonably, consistently, and on schedule.
♦ They test blood glucose levels frequently.
♦ They adjust insulin frequently.

If your child is doing well on his current treatment plan, there may be no need to alter it. But if you would like to see your child achieve better control, you may want to talk with your doctor or diabetes educator about what kind of changes would be right for your child.

THE ROLE OF HEALTH-CARE PROVIDERS

As the parent of a child with diabetes you may encounter several different kinds of health-care providers.

- ◆ A **doctor** who specializes in diabetes can help you make decisions about what kind of insulin your child should take, what dosage regimen works best for your child, and how to handle sick days.
- ◆ A **diabetes educator**, who may be a nurse, can teach you all of the skills you will need to control your child's diabetes and help you learn how to balance food, exercise, and insulin.
- ◆ A **dietitian** can educate you about diet, help you with meal planning, and advise you on the special food needs that children with diabetes have.
- ◆ A **social worker or psychologist** may be able to help you, your child, and your family deal with concerns about living with diabetes.

When these providers work together, they are called a health-care team. The advantage of a health-care team is that you have easy access to several different kinds of help. Health-care teams usually work in big hospitals or special diabetes treatment centers.

If you live a long way from a place that has a health-care team, you may decide to go to your local family doctor for your child's diabetes care. Your doctor may be able to refer you to other health-care providers in your community who can advise you about meal planning, school schedules, insulin adjustments, and coping with stress.

KEEPING YOUR CHILD'S BEST INTERESTS AT HEART

The number one players on the health-care team are, of course, you and your child. When working with your health-care providers (or with other adults in positions of some authority, such as teachers at your child's school), always remember that your child relies on your support.

The following tips may help you to fulfill the role of advocate for your child's needs:

♦ You know your child better than anyone. No one else understands his lifestyle, personality, and likes and dislikes as well as you do. Share what you know about your child openly and honestly with your health-care providers (or your child's teachers). Your child will benefit from your active participation in decisions about his care.

The dietitian included skim milk in 4-year-old Andy's meal plan, but Andy doesn't like milk (especially skim milk). Andy's mother knew he would never drink the milk. She explained the problem honestly to the dietitian. Having this information enabled the dietitian to change Andy's meal plan, replacing the milk with liquids that Andy liked and would drink. This made it easier for both Andy and his mother to follow the meal plan.

♦ Your child depends on you to support him and to speak on his behalf. Very young children often cannot communicate their needs to adults. Older children may have difficulty expressing their real feelings to adults whom they are taught to respect. It's up to you, as a parent and an adult, to communicate on your child's behalf to health-care providers, teachers, and other adults.

Twelve-year-old Missy knew how to give her own insulin injections, but on school mornings when she was in a hurry she relied on her parents to give her insulin. Missy dreaded going for her diabetes checkups because the doctor always told her that at her age she should be giving all of her own injections all the time. Missy felt the doctor just didn't understand, but she had trouble telling the doctor how she felt. When she told her dad what was bothering her, her dad agreed to talk to the doctor. Together, Missy, her dad, and the doctor agreed on a plan: On school mornings Missy and her parents would give her insulin injections on alternate days. In the evenings and on weekends, Missy would do all of her own injections. This experience taught Missy that open and honest communication works best.

♦ Make sure that the goals set for your child's diabetes care are realistic, both for him and for you. A goal is a task that all of the members of the diabetes-care team—especially your child—want to achieve. Goals should be things that everyone agrees are important and that your child can handle successfully.

Fifteen-year-old Joel, who had had diabetes since he was 8, knew he should test his blood glucose four times a day, but he hated doing it. On a good day, he did two blood tests. When Joel wanted to apply for his driver's license, his doctor said that she needed to assess Joel's diabetes control before signing the application. To make the assessment, the doctor needed more blood tests from Joel. Together, Joel, his mother, and the doctor set a goal: Joel would test his blood glucose at least two or three times a day for one month and record the results. At the end of the month, the three of them would look at the test results to assess Joel's diabetes control. Joel could handle this because it took him a step closer to getting something he really wanted—his driver's license.

Everyone who has type I diabetes needs insulin injections because their bodies do not make insulin. If insulin is given by mouth, it is digested like protein and doesn't have any effect on blood glucose levels. The insulin is injected into the fatty tissue under the skin. From there, the insulin is absorbed into the bloodstream.

WHAT KINDS OF INSULIN ARE THERE?

Different kinds of insulin act differently in the body (see charts, pages 16 and 17).

The first insulins came mostly from cows and pigs. Human insulin, which is made in a laboratory, is now widely available and less costly to make than animal insulin. However, animal insulins are still used sometimes, especially in children, because they work for a longer time than human insulins.

If your child is doing well on her current insulin, there may be no need to change. You may, however, want to talk to your doctor about trying another kind of insulin if your child

♦ has wide swings in her blood glucose levels that don't seem to be related to changes in food or exercise

♦ gets redness or swelling in the area where the injection is given

It isn't a good idea to switch insulins without talking to your doctor or diabetes educator about it first.

HOW DO I HANDLE INSULIN?

For general storage, it's a good idea to keep bottles of insulin in the refrigerator (in the butter keeper or somewhere else where it will not freeze). Insulin can break down and not work if it gets too cold (less than 36° F) or too warm (over 86° F).

However, you can carry insulin with you in a purse or backpack. Insulin is stable at room temperature as long as it is stored away from heat and light. If your child uses up a bottle of insulin in less than a month, it's okay to keep it at room temperature. It's a good idea to keep

Types of Insulin

- Different types of insulin work for different periods of time. There are **rapid-acting, intermediate-acting**, and **long-acting** insulins.
- **Rapid-acting** (regular) insulins usually start to work within half an hour after the injection is given. They work best 2 to 5 hours after the injection (this is called the **peak**). Regular insulin is usually given (mixed with intermediate-acting insulin) 30 to 45 minutes before a meal.
- **Intermediate-acting** (NPH or lente) insulins usually work for about 12 to 18 hours. Their peak may be 4 to 15 hours after the injection. This type of insulin is often given in the morning and evening.
- **Long-acting** (ultralente) insulin can work for 18 to 20 hours. It starts to work after 6 to 10 hours and does not peak. It is injected once or twice a day.

the bottle in the carton to protect it from light and keep it clean. Airport X-ray machines do not hurt insulin.

Some people prefer to keep insulin in the refrigerator and take it out for a few minutes to warm up before giving the injection. Other people don't seem to notice if insulin is given cool after being taken straight from the refrigerator.

HOW MUCH INSULIN DOES MY CHILD NEED?

Insulin dosages are based on your child's height, weight, metabolic rate, physical maturity, activity level, and usual diet.

- A heavier or taller child may need more insulin than a smaller child.
- A child who isn't active may need more insulin than one who is active.
- One 12-year-old may take a total morning dose of 30 units while another 12-year-old takes only 20 units.

Taking a larger dose of insulin doesn't mean the child's diabetes is more severe. Different dosages simply mean that children are different.

Your child's need for insulin will change. As children grow, they need to take more insulin. Many children need more insulin in winter than in summer because of differences in their activity level. In winter they are less active and are indoors more. In summer they are outside playing a lot. **Remember: Insulin and exercise lower blood glucose levels. Food increases blood glucose levels.**

Types of Insulin and Their Differences

This list shows the types of insulins available and the differences between them.

Rapid acting (onset 1/2 to 2 hours)

Name	Manufacturer	Form
Humulin R (regular)	Lilly	Human
Iletin I regular	Lilly	Beef/Pork
Iletin II regular	Lilly	Pork
Novolin R (regular)	Novo Nordisk	Human
Novolin R PenFill (regular)	Novo Nordisk	Human
Purified Pork R (regular)	Novo Nordisk	Pork
Velosulin Human (regular) (buffered)	Novo Nordisk	Human

Intermediate acting (onset 2 to 6 hours)

Name	Manufacturer	Form
Humulin L (Lente)	Lilly	Human
Humulin N (NPH)	Lilly	Human
Iletin I Lente	Lilly	Beef/Pork
Iletin I NPH	Lilly	Beef/Pork
Iletin II Lente	Lilly	Pork
Iletin II NPH	Lilly	Pork
Novolin L (Lente)	Novo Nordisk	Human
Novolin N (NPH)	Novo Nordisk	Human
Novolin N PenFill (NPH)	Novo Nordisk	Human
Purified Pork Lente	Novo Nordisk	Pork
Purified Pork N (NPH)	Novo Nordisk	Pork

Long acting (onset 6 to 10 hours)

Name	Manufacturer	Form
Humulin U (Ultralente)	Lilly	Human

Mixtures

Name	Manufacturer	Form
Humulin 50/50 (50% NPH, 50% regular)	Lilly	Human
Humulin 70/30 (70% NPH, 30% regular)	Lilly	Human
Novolin 70/30 (70% NPH, 30% Regular)	Novo Nordisk	Human
Novolin 70/30 PenFill (70% NPH, 30% regular)	Novo Nordisk	Human
Novolin 70/30 Prefilled (70% NPH, 30% regular)	Novo Nordisk	Human

For a few days or months after a child is diagnosed with diabetes, she may need only a very low dose of insulin. During this period, which is sometimes called the "honeymoon period," the child's pancreas is still producing some insulin. However, as time goes by, the insulin-producing cells are being destroyed. Therefore, the body produces less and less insulin. As his body stops making insulin, your child needs more injected insulin.

Big changes in your child's insulin dosage should *only* be made after discussion with your doctor or diabetes educator, but "fine-tuning" your child's dosage from day to day is something you can and should learn to do yourself (see *Adjusting Insulin at Home*, page 31.)

HOW OFTEN DOES MY CHILD NEED INSULIN INJECTIONS?

Most children control diabetes with two or three insulin injections a day. However, some may do best with four injections. The number of daily injections your child needs will depend on several factors:

♦ what type of insulin your child is taking
♦ how able and motivated your child is to care for her diabetes
♦ your child's level of blood glucose control
♦ your child's schedule

Most children take more than one kind of insulin. They may take a rapid-acting insulin (regular) before a meal to balance the intake of food. Before breakfast, and before dinner or at bedtime, they may take an intermediate-acting insulin (NPH or Lente) that works for a longer time. (See the chart of different types of insulin on page 17.)

Rapid-acting insulin is usually given 30 to 45 minutes before a meal. To avoid gaps or overlaps between doses, a good rule of thumb is to always give the injections at regular times, within about an hour (see chart on scheduling meals and insulin injections, page 19).

A new type of extremely rapid-acting insulin is expected to become available sometime in 1996. Because this insulin goes to work as soon as it is injected, there is no need to wait to eat a meal after taking it. When this new type of insulin becomes available, it will add more flexibility to diabetes care.

During summer vacation and at other times when your child's schedule changes, it's okay to alter the times of insulin injections. For example, if your child wants to get up and eat breakfast later during the summer months, the whole schedule can be pushed

Scheduling Meals and Insulin Injections

A helpful rule of thumb is to always give injections and have meals at the same time give or take an hour. Here's how this might work:

Usual getting-up time: 7 a.m.
♦ Give injection of intermediate-acting insulin no earlier than 6 a.m. and no later than 8 a.m.

Usual lunch time: Noon
♦ Eat lunch no earlier than 11 a.m. and no later than 1 p.m. If your child takes rapid-acting (regular) insulin, give the injection 30 minutes before lunch if possible.

Usual dinner time: 5 p.m.
♦ Give injection of intermediate-acting or rapid-acting (regular) insulin no earlier than 4 p.m. and no later than 6 p.m.

back. Your doctor or diabetes educator can help you decide how to handle these kinds of schedule changes.

Some children follow a regimen called multiple daily injections (MDI). They get one or two injections of intermediate- or long-acting insulin every day, plus an injection of rapid-acting insulin before each meal or snack.

The MDI regimen tries to mimic the way a normal pancreas works. Multiple injections provide a bit more flexibility: The insulin dosage can be adjusted frequently during the day according to food intake and activity level. You may want to ask your doctor or diabetes educator whether an MDI regimen would be right for your child.

MDI is a form of intensive diabetes management where the aim is to keep blood glucose levels as close to normal as possible all the time.

GIVING THE INJECTIONS

Giving your child an insulin injection can be hard, both emotionally and physically, especially if your child is young and squirms a lot. The charts on giving insulin injections (page 24) and making insulin injections easier (pages 25 and 26) may give you some guidance.

How to Draw Up One Type of Insulin

1. Wash your hands thoroughly.

2. Select the injection site according to your rotation schedule (see *What Is Site Rotation?* page 24).

3. Clean the injection site with soap and water or alcohol. (Alcohol may be used if it is more convenient, but it dries the skin.)

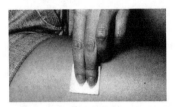

4. Gently roll the insulin bottle between your hands to mix the insulin. Wipe the top of the insulin bottle with alcohol.

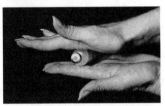

5. Draw back the plunger on the syringe to the correct number of insulin units.

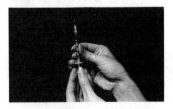
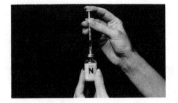

6. Holding the insulin bottle upright, insert the needle into the bottle and push the plunger in. This injects air into the bottle.

7. Keeping the needle in the bottle, turn the bottle upside down and slowly pull back the plunger until the syringe has more insulin in it than you need.

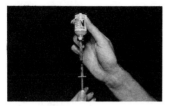

8. Gently tap the syringe to move air bubbles to the top.

9. With the needle still in the bottle, slowly press the plunger forward to expel the air bubbles and extra insulin.

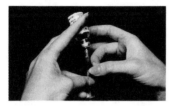

10. Double-check that you have the correct number of insulin units in the syringe.

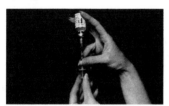

11. Gently pull the needle out of the bottle.

How to Draw Up Two Types of Insulin

1. Wash your hands thoroughly.

2. Select the injection site according to your rotation schedule (see *What Is Site Rotation?* page 24).

3. Clean the injection site with soap and water or alcohol. (Alcohol may be used if it is more convenient, but it dries the skin.)

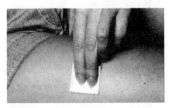

4. Gently roll the insulin bottles between your hands to mix the insulin. Wipe the top of the insulin bottle with alcohol.

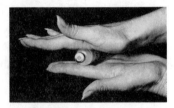

5. Draw back the plunger on the syringe to the correct number of units of rapid-acting (clear) insulin to be given.

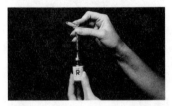

6. Holding the bottle of rapid-acting insulin upright, insert the needle into the air space in the bottle and push the plunger in. This injects air into the bottle. Remove the needle.

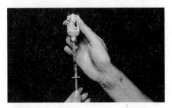

7. Draw back the plunger on the syringe to the correct number of units of intermediate-acting (cloudy) insulin to be given.

8. Holding the bottle of intermediate-acting insulin upright, insert the needle into the bottle and push the plunger in. This injects air into the bottle.

9. Keeping the needle in the bottle, turn the bottle of intermediate-acting insulin upside down and slowly pull back the plunger until the syringe has more insulin in it than you need.

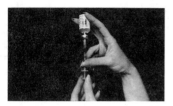

10. Gently tap the syringe to move air bubbles to the top.

11. With the needle still in the bottle, slowly press the plunger forward to expel the air bubbles and extra insulin.

12. Double-check that you have the correct number of units of intermediate-acting insulin in the syringe.

13. Gently pull the needle out of the bottle of intermediate-acting insulin.

14. Insert the needle into the bottle of rapid-acting insulin and slowly withdraw the correct number of units. *Take care that none of the intermediate-acting insulin already in the syringe is pushed into the bottle of rapid-acting insulin. If the insulins are accidentally mixed in the bottle, you must discard the bottle of rapid-acting insulin because it may not act rapidly any more.*

15. Check for air bubbles in the syringe. If there is a large air bubble in the syringe after you have added the rapid-acting insulin, discard the syringe and start again. If there is a small air bubble that can be tapped out without noticeably changing the dosage, go ahead and give the injection. Small air bubbles will not harm your child, but they can alter the amount of insulin injected.

The advantage of drawing up the intermediate-acting (cloudy) insulin first and then the rapid-acting (clear) insulin is that you can see your mistake immediately if you accidentally push cloudy insulin into the bottle of clear insulin. Another way of doing it would be to draw up the rapid-acting (clear) insulin first. This lessens the risk of contaminating the bottle of rapid-acting insulin.

How to Give the Insulin Injection

♦ With one hand, gently pinch up the skin in the area where you are giving the injection. (This avoids injecting the insulin into a muscle, which can be painful and can also alter the way insulin is absorbed by the body.)
♦ With the other hand, hold the syringe like a pencil.
♦ Insert the needle gently at a 90° angle to the skin.
♦ Push gently but steadily on the plunger.
♦ Ask your child if she prefers you to give the injection quickly or slowly.
♦ Pull the needle out and throw it immediately (uncapped) into a proper disposal container (a "sharps box")
♦ After the injection, praise your child for doing a good job and give her a big hug.

WHAT IS SITE ROTATION?

Giving your child's insulin injections in different places is called site rotation. It's a good idea to do this because always giving injections in the same place may cause puffy, lumpy spots. Injecting into these lumps (or into scar tissue) can slow down insulin action.

When insulin is injected, it can attract fat into the injection area, leading to the formation of lumps made of fat and scar tissue. These lumps can affect the way insulin is absorbed. If insulin is poorly absorbed, your child may have wide swings in blood glucose levels.

Insulin is absorbed most quickly when the injection is given in the abdomen. It is absorbed a bit more slowly when the injection is given in the arms, more slowly still in the legs, and slowest of all when the injection is given in the hip.

Having a plan for rotating where you give your child's injections can help to make sure that insulin is absorbed at the same rate. For example, if your child gets two injections a day, you could give the morning injection in an arm and the evening injection in a leg. Or you could give the morning injection in the left arm and the evening injection in the right arm.

You may also want to rotate within one area–like the fleshy part of the upper arm–by dividing it with imaginary lines (see *Where to Give the Injections*, pages 28 and 29).

How you rotate is less important than doing it. Rotating injections according to a plan also helps you and your child to

Tips for Easier Insulin Injections—Part I

If you are worried that the injection hurts your child:
◆ Give yourself an injection with an empty syringe (do not inject air) to see what the needle feels like. (Or get someone—perhaps your child—to give you the injection.) You may be relieved to find that it hardly hurts at all because the needle is so fine.

If your child wants to give her own injection in the arm:
◆ Press the arm against a chair or a wall or over a bent knee to help to make the fleshy part of the arm stand out.

If insulin frequently leaks out after you give the injection:
◆ Try pulling the skin to one side when pinching it up. When you finish giving the injection and release the skin, it will cover up the needle mark and prevent leaking.
◆ After pushing in the plunger, count slowly to 10 before removing the needle.

If the plunger won't push in easily:
◆ Pull back slightly on the needle. If the plunger still won't move easily, take the needle out and try giving the injection at another spot.
◆ If the plunger still won't move, fill a new syringe and start over. The insulin may be jamming the needle.

remember where the right place for the injection is each time. If your child is having wide swings in blood glucose, keeping track of where you give the injections can help you to see if the swings have a pattern that is related to the injection site. (For example, do your child's blood glucose levels swing more when the injections are given in the hip than when they are given in the arms?)

Your doctor or diabetes educator can help you and your child decide on the best way to do site rotation.

HOW CAN I HELP MY CHILD TO ACCEPT INSULIN INJECTIONS?
Every child is different. Some children adjust well to insulin injections, while others find them very hard to accept. There are several reasons why a child may protest or fight injections.
◆ The injection may be painful.
◆ The child may be expressing anger about having diabetes.
◆ The child may be afraid of needles.

25

Tips for Easier Insulin Injections—Part II

If your child gets bruising around the area of the injection:
♦ Bruising is usually caused by a broken small blood vessel. It's hard to avoid bruising once in a while. Unless it happens a lot, it isn't something you should worry about. If it does happen a lot, check to see whether it's happening at all injection sites or mostly at one site (such as the arms). Ask your nurse educator for help with your injection technique.

If the area of the injection turns red:
♦ Redness may be caused by alcohol that is used to clean the skin. If you use alcohol, allow it to dry thoroughly before giving the injection. If alcohol irritates your child's skin, use soap and water instead.
♦ Rarely, redness may be caused by an allergic reaction to insulin. (If your child is taking human insulin, allergic reactions are **extremely** rare.) The spot may be tender or itchy. If your child's injection sites turn red or itchy, tell your doctor about it.

If the injection is painful:
♦ An injection may be more painful than usual if:
  – it is given in dense muscle tissue
  – it caused a bruise
  – the injection was given close to a nerve ending
  – the needle is accidentally blunted when the insulin is withdrawn from the bottle
  – the needle is inserted too slowly as it goes through the skin
  Consult your doctor or diabetes educator if your child frequently complains of pain during injections. However, many children complain more at the idea of having the injection than because the injection is painful.
♦ An injection aid (injector) may help. Injectors can make it easier to put the needle through the skin or to give injections in hard-to-reach places. *Jet injectors* use a pressurized stream of air instead of a needle to inject the insulin. Your doctor or diabetes educator can give you more information about injection aids.

♦ It may be an age-related problem. For example, preschool children generally do not do well with any kind of intrusive procedure.

You may find it helpful to use an injection aid—see *Tips for Easier Injections* (page 25 and this page). Going over how to give injections with your diabetes educator may also help.

Very young children may fuss during injections. It may help to tell your child that the injection keeps her healthy and to give her a big hug when it's over. The fuss usually subsides over time as your child becomes used to getting injections regularly.

To get your child used to the idea of getting insulin injections, it may help in the beginning to try to associate the injection with something the child enjoys, like watching a favorite show on television: "Every day, just before you watch XYZ show, mom (or dad) will give you an injection to keep you well."

In families where both parents are available, it's a good idea for both to be involved in giving your child's insulin injections. That way, both parents share the responsibility and each can get a break.

It's normal for children to protest about injections at times, especially when they are tired, stressed, or unhappy. However, if your family's life is consistently disrupted by your child's resistance to injections, a social worker or psychologist may be able to help with a plan to smooth things out (see *Asking for Help*, page 109).

WHEN IS MY CHILD READY TO GIVE HER OWN INJECTIONS?

Learning to give their own injections is an important step for children with diabetes because it helps them be more independent. They can go to visit relatives or on sleepovers with friends.

There is no strict rule about when children are ready to start giving their own injections. One child may be ready to do it (with a parent watching) at age 7 while another child may not be ready until age 12. The right age for your child is whenever she is capable of doing it and when both you and the child feel comfortable about her doing it.

Try to be patient and let the child do the injections when she feels ready, but remind her that you are always there to help. She may quickly get the hang of giving her own injections and may do it without your help at all for a while. Then, for some reason, she may again want you to help or to give the injection. It is common for children to move forward and then step back. Sometimes they need reassurance that they can still rely on their parents' support.

Your child may feel okay about giving injections in the legs but not in the arms or abdomen. You may need to keep doing

Where to Give the Injections

Where to give the injections on your child's arm:

♦ Ask your child to put her left hand, on her right arm by the shoulder, with her fingers closed (Figure A). The bottom of the hand is the highest point where injections should be given.

♦ Next, ask your child to grab her arm just above the right elbow (Figure B). The top of the hand is the lowest point where injections should be given.

♦ In the space between your child's hands, draw two imaginary lines down the arm–one down the side and one down the middle of the back of the arm.

♦ Give the injections along these two tracks, measuring from one spot to the next by the width of two of your child's fingers.

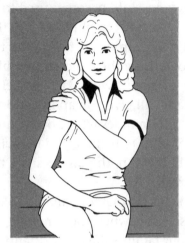

Figure A

Where to give the injections on your child's thigh:

♦ Ask your child to put one hand at the top of her thigh (by the hip) and the other hand on top of her knee on the same leg (Figure C). It's okay to give injections in the space between the hands.

♦ Draw three imaginary lines, one down the top of the leg and one on each side–one toward the outside and one toward the inside.

♦ Give the injections along these three tracks, measuring from one spot to the next by the width of two of your child's fingers.

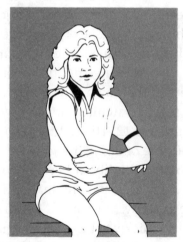

Figure B

Where to give the injections on your child's abdomen:

♦ Draw an imaginary one-inch circle around your child's navel. Don't give injections inside the circle because this area can be tender.

♦ Give the injections in the surrounding area of the abdomen, stomach, and hip.

Where to give the injections in your child's hip:

♦ The upper outer quadrant of the buttock (actually the hip) is a suitable place for injections, although it may be a difficult area for your child to reach to give her own injections. Check with your child's doctor for instructions on giving injections in the hip (Figure D).

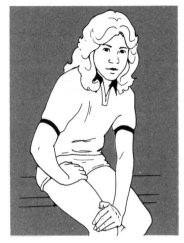

Figure C

If your child gets puffiness or lumps near the area of an injection:

♦ Don't give any more injections in that spot for 3 to 6 months. The lumps should go away.

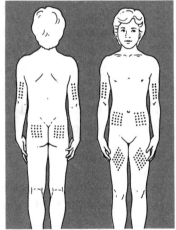

Figure D

Encouraging Your Child to do Her Own Injections

Encourage your child a step at a time to take responsibility for giving her own insulin injections.

♦ Start by asking your child to choose the injection site, to clean the site, or to prepare the dose.
♦ Then suggest that your child push in the plunger or take the needle out of the skin after the injection.
♦ As your child becomes more comfortable doing these things, suggest that she hold the syringe.
♦ Give your child lots of praise as she takes on greater responsibility for injections.
♦ Eventually, your child will be able to do the whole procedure herself!

those injections for a while. Or you may want to suggest that you give the injections on odd-numbered days and that your child gives them on even-numbered days.

Wanting to go on a camping trip or sleep at a friend's house may give your child an incentive to learn to do her own injections. Getting to know other children who can give their own injections may also help. Encourage your child to attend a youth group or a camp for children with diabetes. And don't be surprised if a letter home from camp announces with pride, "I gave my own injection today!" (See *Should I Send My Child to Diabetes Camp?* page 92.)

Even when you feel comfortable about your child giving her own injections, supervision is recommended. A responsible adult should check to make sure the dose is correct and that all the insulin is injected. Children (even teenagers) always feel more secure when their parents are involved in their diabetes care.

REUSING DISPOSABLE SYRINGES

In the past, people with diabetes were taught to throw away disposable syringes after one use. These days, however, many people reuse syringes to save money. It's okay to reuse syringes as long as you are careful (see *Reusing Syringes Safely*, page 31). Repeated use of syringes has not been shown to cause infections or other problems. However, the needle can become dull with repeated use.

Reusing Syringes Safely

◆ Discuss the pros and cons and safety rules of syringe reuse with your health-care provider before doing it.

◆ Recap the needle with a one-handed scoop-up method. (With the syringe in your hand, scoop up the cap as it lies on the table.)

◆ The needle and syringe may be stored in the refrigerator or another safe place.

◆ Do not clean the needle with alcohol. A silicon coating on the needle helps to make the injection less painful. Cleaning the needle with alcohol may remove this coating.

◆ Do not reuse bent needles or syringes that have fallen on the floor.

◆ **Never** share syringes.

Many people with diabetes will use one syringe each day, recapping it after each use. **It's very important that no one else use an already used syringe.** Sharing used syringes can spread viruses that cause hepatitis and AIDS.

Disposing of needles

It's important to handle and dispose of used needles and lancets safely. Unless you reuse syringes, do not recap needles or lancets. This helps you avoid being accidently stuck. Your diabetes educator may be able to get you a special box to use for disposing of needles and lancets. Otherwise, use a plastic milk carton or a soda bottle. Check with your local trash disposal company to find out how to label and dispose of the used needle container.

ADJUSTING INSULIN AT HOME

Your child's insulin needs vary from day to day. With help from your doctor or nurse educator, you can learn how to make small adjustments in your child's daily insulin dosage depending on what she has to eat and how active she is.

"Fine-tuning" your child's dosage helps to keep her blood glucose levels in the target range. Looking for patterns in glucose levels will help you to adjust the insulin dose. Don't be afraid to make small adjustments. Making adjustments shows that you are working with your child's blood glucose levels. (See *The Nitty-Gritty*

3—Meal Planning and *Playing Games and Sports Safely* for more on how food and exercise affect your child's need for insulin.)

Remember that big changes in your child's insulin dose should only be made with the guidance of your doctor or diabetes educator. If your child has a lot of blood glucose readings outside of the target range, talk to your doctor. This may mean you'll need to change her insulin dosages, food, or activity schedule.

Remember, too, that neither the amount of insulin nor the number of injections your child needs is a measure of the severity of her diabetes. As your child grows, she will need more insulin. The diabetes hasn't gotten worse—your child got bigger!

How do food and exercise affect my child's insulin needs?

The amount of insulin your child needs from day to day is affected by how much and what food she eats and how active she is. Your diabetes educator can help you learn how to make daily adjustments to your child's insulin dosage depending on the food and activities planned for that day.

Food raises blood glucose while exercise lowers it. Eating more than usual or eating a sugar-rich food like birthday cake can make your child's blood glucose rise. Taking part in a strenuous game can make it drop.

Extra food helps to balance exercise. When your child is going to exercise, you can decrease insulin, give her more food to eat, or both. When blood glucose runs high, you can give more insulin or adjust the child's meal plan so she is eating less. If your child is going through a phase when she is eating less than usual, she will need less insulin.

> Stacey is on the high school swim team. She has swim practice every day at 3 p.m. She has a snack before practice, but she doesn't want to eat a lot of food right before swimming. However, she also doesn't want to start feeling "low" while she's in the pool. In the morning, Stacey takes intermediate-acting (NPH) insulin, which is working at peak effectiveness at about 3 p.m. To prevent a "low" during swim practice, Stacey reduces her NPH dose by 2 units.

Your doctor or diabetes educator can help you to understand how to balance food, activity, and insulin to keep your child's blood glucose level in the target range. For more about using food to balance insulin, see *The Nitty-Gritty 3—Meal Planning*.

How do I fine-tune my child's dosage?

Fine-tuning your child's insulin dosage means:

♦ learning to look for patterns of high or low blood glucose

♦ trying to figure out why high or low blood glucose levels occur

♦ adjusting your child's insulin dose, food, or timing of meals to fix the problem.

If your child's blood glucose level is a bit too high, you can *increase* the insulin dose or reduce food. If your child's blood glucose level is a bit too low, you can *decrease* the dose or add food. When glucose is:

High ➡ Increase insulin

Low ➡ Decrease insulin

However, there are some exceptions to this rule (see *Rebound*, page 70).

James, who is 11 years old, is going on a scout camp overnight trip. When James is camping, his glucose levels are usually in the good range because of all the games and activities. But the troop is planning to roast marshmallows and make popcorn at the campfire. James wants to eat the marshmallows with his friends, but they will probably raise his glucose level.

His mom suggests that he test his blood glucose before the campfire. She tells him that his glucose level will probably be okay from all of the games played that evening. She writes the following note for James:

Dear James,

　　Eat 4 to 6 cups of popcorn.

　　Eat 6 marshmallows if your blood test is less than 80.

　　Eat 4 marshmallows if your blood test is 80 to 180.

　　Eat 2 marshmallows if your blood test is over 180.

　　　　　　　　Love,

　　　　　　　　Mom

Adjustment Scale for Regular Insulin

Find your child's blood glucose range in the column on the left. Then look at the column on the right to find the corresponding insulin dose. For example, if Suzie's blood glucose reading is 142 mg/dl, she should take 5 units of insulin.

Subtract 2 units if your child will be exercising. For example, if Jimmy's blood glucose reading is 135 mg/dl but he will be playing soccer after school, he should take 3 units of insulin.

Blood glucose reading (mg/dl) before breakfast:	Regular insulin dose:
< 70	3 units
70–120	4 units
121–180	5 units
181–240	6 units
241–300	7 units
> 301	8 units

Seven-year-old Ashleigh is going to a birthday party from 6 to 8 p.m. The party theme is a "tea party," with very little activity planned. Ashleigh wants to enjoy the birthday cake that will be served at the party. Cake always makes her glucose levels high. Ashleigh gets regular insulin every day before dinner at 5 p.m. Her mother gives her an extra unit of regular insulin with her predinner injection on the day of the party. Ashleigh can now enjoy the birthday cake and still prevent her glucose levels from going too high.

The chart on this page gives an example of how insulin doses can be adjusted according to what the blood glucose level is. Your doctor or diabetes educator can prepare a dosage adjustment chart or scale that's right for your child.

Why are patterns in blood glucose levels important?

It may take a few days for a dosage adjustment to make a difference in your child's blood glucose control. So it's important to look for *patterns* in blood glucose levels over periods of two to three days.

Like most children, your child probably takes more than one type of insulin. For example, she may take a mixture of intermediate-acting (NPH) and rapid-acting (regular) insulin in the morning, regular insulin before dinner, and NPH before her bedtime snack. This means that at different times of day a different type of insulin is working in your child's body.

Knowing what is causing a problem, as well as what time of day a problem is occurring, can help you decide how to fine-tune your child's dosage. This is why blood glucose testing throughout the day is so important (see the next chapter for more about blood glucose testing).

Mike had soccer practice from 7 to 8 p.m. on Mondays, Wednesdays, and Fridays. Halfway through practice he would get symptoms of low blood glucose. To prevent low blood glucose during soccer practice, Mike reduced his before-dinner dose of regular insulin by 2 units on soccer nights.

WHAT IS AN INSULIN PUMP?

An insulin pump works by mimicking the way insulin normally works in the body. The pump is connected to a tiny needle inserted in the abdomen. The needle stays in place for several days. The pump itself can be attached to a belt. It delivers a steady, low dose of regular insulin to the body all day and all night. The dose can be increased to give extra insulin before a meal.

An insulin pump requires care to prevent infection and ensure proper functioning. A person who is using a pump needs to test blood glucose at least four times a day. Using a pump means working closely with a doctor or nurse to decide on insulin dosages and to handle any problems that come up. For example, the needle site may become infected, the tubing may leak, or the needle may become plugged up.

Is a pump right for my child?

Some people with diabetes have found the insulin pump to be very helpful. Using a pump means they no longer need insulin injections. The pump keeps their blood glucose levels close to normal all the time.

Using a pump may be an option for a child or teenager who
♦ wants a more flexible meal plan or freedom from multiple insulin injections
♦ is mature enough to look after the pump and check her blood glucose levels regularly
♦ recognizes the signs and symptoms of low blood glucose and knows how to treat them when they occur.

Using an insulin pump is a form of intensive diabetes management, where the aim is to keep blood glucose levels as close to normal as possible all the time.

If your child is interested in using an insulin pump, you should arrange to see a doctor and a diabetes educator who have experience looking after people who use pumps.

Regular testing of blood glucose levels is a very important part of your child's diabetes care. It's the only way to know if your child's blood glucose level is in the target range. Glucose testing means using a meter to measure the amount of glucose in a drop of capillary blood, usually from a finger. Blood is placed on a glucose-sensitive test strip or pad and inserted into a glucose meter. Glucose meters are so easy to use that children can quickly learn how to do their own glucose tests.

Knowing your child's blood glucose level before a meal can help you to decide whether to encourage him to eat an extra helping of food or to give more or less than the usual insulin dose at the next injection.

As discussed in *The Nitty-Gritty 1—Insulin Treatment*, learning to look for patterns in your child's blood glucose levels will help you to fine-tune his insulin dosages, activity level, and food intake. Your doctor or diabetes educator can help you to do this.

HOW OFTEN SHOULD MY CHILD'S BLOOD GLUCOSE BE TESTED?

How often your child's blood glucose level needs to be tested depends on your child's needs. His age, eating habits, activity level, and insulin needs, as well as how quickly he is growing, all need to be considered in determining how frequently he needs to test.

Four blood glucose tests a day are usually recommended for children and teens. If testing at school is very disruptive to your child or to his class, a lunchtime test may not be necessary. However, children on multiple daily injections or an insulin pump will need to test at least four times a day.

Frequent blood glucose tests are especially important in very young children who can't talk because they can't tell you whether they are feeling symptoms of low or high blood glucose. **When in doubt—test!**

Other times to do blood glucose tests

Your doctor may sometimes ask you to test your child's blood glucose levels at other times of day than when you usually do it. This can help you to get a clearer picture of what happens to your child's glucose levels throughout the day.

Doing the Fingerstick

1. Wash the child's hands with warm soapy water and dry well.
2. Prepare your meter and test strip according to the manufacturer's instructions.
3. Choose the spot where you are going to do the fingerstick.
4. Place the finger-pricking device on the side of the finger. Press the release mechanism.
5. Squeeze out a large "hanging" drop of blood. If you have a hard time drawing a drop of blood, try this:
   ◆ after sticking the finger, hang the hand down and gently shake it
   ◆ lightly squeeze the finger, moving from the middle joint toward the fingertip (this is called "milking" the finger)
6. Place the blood as directed in the instructions for your meter.
7. Wait for the results. Record the number in your daily log.

Tips For Easier, Less Painful Fingersticks

◆ New finger-pricking devices and fine lances are available that are light and easy to handle and that make doing the fingerstick almost painless. Some of these devices are specially made for children's sensitive fingers. They go deep enough into the skin to draw a drop of blood but not deep enough to hurt much or leave much of a mark. Ask your diabetes educator or pharmacist to tell you about these devices.
◆ Prick the sides of the fingers to draw blood. The sides have a good blood supply and fewer nerve endings than the fingertips.
◆ In young children with tiny fingers, you can also do fingersticks in the earlobes, heels, and toes. (In infants, it is safest to use the outer sides of the heels.)

For example, blood glucose levels may always be normal before meals. But how do you know whether they shoot up right after meals? The way to find out is to sometimes do a test an hour or two after a meal. Your doctor will tell you whether this test should be an extra one or whether it should be done instead of one of the usual tests.

You can use the additional information you get from these tests to help you make decisions about your child's daily food intake and his exercise and insulin routine.

It can also be helpful to check blood glucose after your child eats a food that you suspect raises his glucose level unusually high. This can help you to decide whether to give extra insulin. Extra blood tests when your child is sick can help you decide how to adjust insulin dosages and food. Any time that your child acts like or claims to feel like his blood glucose is low, it's a good idea to do a blood test. This can prevent "anxiety eating" when a child mistakes nervousness for low blood glucose.

Checking blood glucose is helpful before, during, and after exercise. If your child's blood glucose is on the low side before exercise, you can see that he eats an extra snack. Doing a check during exercise can tell a youngster if sweating and a pounding heart are caused by exertion or by low blood glucose. (See *Playing Games and Sports Safely*.)

RECORDING RESULTS OF BLOOD GLUCOSE TESTS

Each time you do a blood glucose test, it's very important to record the reading. A log book will help you to keep track of this information. Most log books have a comments section for recording events during the day, such as exercise, meal times, special treats eaten, low blood glucose symptoms, or illness. This log can help you to detect patterns and trends in glucose levels. There is a sample log on page 40.

HOW DO I KNOW IF I'M TESTING BLOOD GLUCOSE CORRECTLY?

The new blood glucose meters make testing pretty easy to do. Most meters are designed to make sure they are working properly. Your health-care provider can teach you how to do blood glucose testing correctly and answer any questions that you may have. In addition, the manufacturers of meters always have service departments that you can call with questions or concerns.

Remember to take your meter and your book of written records with you when you go to see your health-care provider. He or she may want to check the meter to make sure it is working right. Your doctor or diabetes educator can also help you to look for patterns in your child's blood glucose readings and decide whether your child's insulin dose needs to be changed.

MAKING SURE YOUR METER IS ACCURATE

Every brand of meter allows you to check its accuracy so that you know your results are true. This is done with a check strip, a

Diabetes Weekly Diary

Month: _____ **Year:** _____

Insulin (Brand, Type, Species) _____

Date/Day	Insulin Dose					Blood Glucose and Urine Ketone Test Results							
	Time / Units					Breakfast		Lunch	Dinner	Bedtime / Night		Comments/Exercise/Injection Sites
						Urine	Blood	Blood	Blood	Blood		

control solution, or both. A check strip should read a certain glucose level when inserted. You use a control solution as a substitute for blood. This solution has a certain amount of glucose in it. Control solutions are made to work with the brand of meter they are sold for, so be sure not to cross brands. The results you get with the check strip or control solution should be within a certain range. If on testing you find that your meter is out of the accepted range for accuracy, call the technical services phone number for your brand of meter.

Another way of checking the accuracy of your meter is to compare a sample of blood on your meter with a laboratory result for the blood. This works best when the same sample of blood is used for both. This needs to be done when you visit your health-care provider, because you will use blood taken from a vein rather than from the capillaries in the finger. Glucose results from capillary blood are about 11% higher than with blood from a vein. If the reading from your meter and the result from the laboratory are within 20% of each other, your meter is accurate.

URINE TESTING

Urine testing can be a useful way of telling if blood glucose levels have been high, especially overnight. If your child's blood glucose level is normal in the morning but there is a lot of glucose in his urine, it's likely that his glucose level ran high sometime during the night. However, urine glucose testing is not a substitute for blood glucose testing.

Urine testing to check for **ketones** is very important. Ketones are by-products of fat breakdown that can appear in the urine when your child

♦ has a viral illness
♦ has not taken enough insulin
♦ is under a lot of emotional stress
♦ is not eating well
♦ has recently had an episode of low blood glucose

Test your child's urine for ketones every morning. When your child is sick, test for ketones every time he urinates. Tell your doctor or nurse if you find a large amount of ketones in your child's urine or if ketones are present (even in small amounts) on more than one test. Ask your doctor for more specific guidance on who to call and what to do when you find ketones in your child's urine.

Ketones can cause the blood to become acidic, which leads to nausea, vomiting, and flu-like symptoms. Large amounts of ketones in the urine can lead to **ketoacidosis.** (See *Ketoacidosis,* page 69.)

GETTING YOUR CHILD TO TEST REGULARLY

Getting your child to do urine ketone testing once a day and blood glucose testing three or more times a day can be a challenge. Your child may resist testing because he does not feel it is important or doesn't want to get bad news. At times your child may find it hard to do the testing himself, and you may have to take over for a while.

Giving praise each time a test is done or awarding stars or points toward an extra privilege or special "fun" event can help to get your child to test regularly. In time, the need for these kinds of "carrots" usually fades away, but continual positive reinforcement remains important. Let your child know that even high test results give you the information you need to help him control blood glucose.

WHAT IS THE GLYCATED HEMOGLOBIN (HbA$_1$) TEST?

This is a useful blood test that your doctor should do to measure your child's average blood glucose control over a period of a couple of months.

The test measures **glycated hemoglobin (HbA$_1$ or HbA$_{1c}$)**. Hemoglobin is a substance in red blood cells. HbA is a type of hemoglobin to which glucose attaches. If your child's blood glucose is high, the level of HbA will be high too. Because you can't affect the results of the HbA test by last-minute efforts at control, the test acts as a check on true glucose control over a several-month period.

The HbA$_1$ test was one of the tools used in the Diabetes Control and Complications Trial (see page 9). One of the things doctors tried to do in this study was to get patients' HbA levels as close to normal as possible. This can be hard to do, especially in children and teenagers. But we now know that keeping HbA levels close to normal may help to delay or prevent complications of diabetes. (See *Complications of Diabetes*, page 76.)

> Sam's blood glucose test records looked as though his glucose level was in the target range most of the time, but the HbA test results were high. This told the doctor that Sam may not be testing at the times his blood glucose readings are high, or that there could be a problem with the way Sam or his parents do blood glucose testing or record test results.

Food is a very important part of our lives. We need food to survive, of course, but eating is also a very important ritual. Many families enjoy sitting down to a meal together every day. We celebrate birthdays, sporting events, and holidays with food. Certain foods have special meaning for us, like pumpkin pie at Thanksgiving or popcorn at the movies.

As the parent of a child with diabetes, you probably have many questions and concerns about what your child can eat. How can you meet your child's dietary needs without disrupting meals for the rest of the family? How can you be sure that she always eats the right foods? Can she eat pumpkin pie or birthday cake?

You do need to pay close attention to what your child eats and when she eats. Food raises your child's blood glucose levels. Meal planning helps you to balance food, insulin, and exercise. But your family *can* continue to enjoy meals—every day *and* on special occasions. A healthy diet for your child with diabetes is a healthy diet for your whole family.

WHY IS MEAL PLANNING IMPORTANT?

Meal planning for children with diabetes is important for two reasons:

♦ It helps to make sure that your child gets the right amount of calories and nutrients to grow and develop normally.

♦ It helps to control your child's blood glucose levels.

Your child's need for nutrients from food depends on her age, sex, weight, and activity level. As your child grows, her food needs change. Having a meal plan helps you adjust to these changes. It's a good idea to go over your child's meal plan once a year with your dietitian to make sure the plan is still right for your child.

HOW DOES A MEAL PLAN WORK?

Every child's meal plan is different. It depends on what kinds of food your child likes or dislikes, as well as on her age, weight, and so on. Generally, however, any meal plan for a child with diabetes does the following things:

- ◆ It helps to make sure your child eats a balanced diet.
- ◆ It includes three meals and two or three snacks a day and sets times of day when meals and snacks should usually be eaten.
- ◆ It limits the amount of fat, cholesterol, and sugar that your child eats.
- ◆ It helps to control your child's diabetes by balancing food with insulin to keep blood glucose levels within a target range. This balance includes matching insulin doses to the amount of food to be eaten and insulin action times to eating times.

Having a dietitian as a member of your health-care team is very helpful when it comes to meal planning. The dietitian can answer questions or concerns that you or your child may have.

LET APPETITE BE YOUR GUIDE

A child's appetite varies widely and usually indicates the need for food. During growth spurts or times of lots of physical activity, your child may eat hardy. Other times, you may wonder how she keeps going on so little food. Yet, this is the way children normally eat, and having diabetes doesn't change it. You will need to learn how to make changes in insulin dose based on your child's appetite. It is also important to make meal times pleasant, which means avoiding a battle of wills over food.

When your child was diagnosed with diabetes, she may have lost weight or perhaps not gained weight for a while. Once treatment begins, she may have a tremendous appetite and eat well. After the weight is made up, she will not want so much food. Your dietitian will give you a meal plan at diagnosis, but you may need to increase or decrease the number of calories to keep up with her appetite. Therefore, you'll to keep in touch with your dietitian when making meal plan changes and deciding how much insulin to give to balance the food.

If she's hungry, you can give your child extra food, but do it *at meal times*. Try to avoid giving extra between meal snacks. Give your child seconds on foods from all food groups, not just potatoes or bread. On the other hand, if she does not eat well at a meal, try giving a drink such as milk or juice to help keep her blood glucose levels up until the next meal.

A BALANCED DIET

Most people have heard of the "four food groups." These days most food experts suggest dividing foods into five groups instead of four:

♦ grains and breads
♦ milk and dairy products
♦ fruits and vegetables
♦ meat and meat substitutes
♦ fats and sweets

The three major nutrients our bodies get from food are carbohydrates, protein, and fat. These nutrients do different things in the body.

♦ Carbohydrates are the body's main source of energy. They are found in fruits, vegetables, bread, cereal, milk, rice, potatoes, and pasta. These foods are turned into glucose during digestion fairly quickly, which increases the blood glucose level fairly quickly.

♦ Protein is used to build and repair body tissue. It is found in meat, poultry, fish, eggs, cheese, peanut butter, and milk. Proteins digest into glucose about half as fast as carbohydrate, causing a slower rise in the blood glucose level that lasts longer.

♦ Fat provides reserves of energy. It is found in marbled meat, the skin of poultry, whole milk, butter, cheese, and oils (corn oil, olive oil, etc.). It is difficult for the body to turn fat into glucose. Fat has little effect on the blood glucose level other than slowing down the digestion of other nutrients.

If your child eats a variety of foods, vitamin and mineral supplements are not necessary.

In scientific studies, diets high in fat have been shown to increase people's risk of getting diseases like high blood pressure and heart disease. People with diabetes generally have a higher risk than other people of getting heart disease later in life. Eating less fat helps to reduce the risk of developing these problems.

Healthy eating guidelines developed by the U.S. government advise Americans to cut the fat in their diets to no more than 30 percent of all calories they eat. The Food Guide Pyramid (see next page) was invented to help people make healthy food choices.

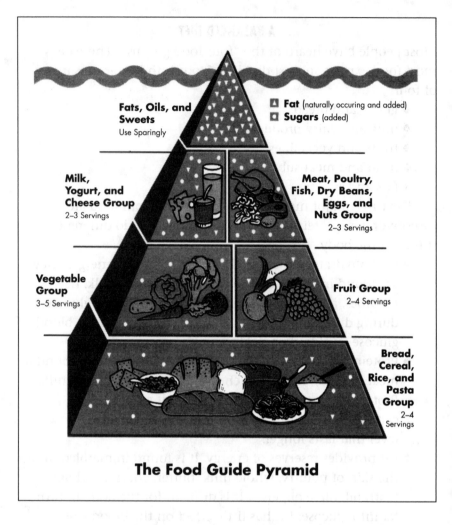

Fat (naturally occuring and added)
Sugars (added)

Fats, Oils, and Sweets
Use Sparingly

Milk, Yogurt, and Cheese Group
2–3 Servings

Meat, Poultry, Fish, Dry Beans, Eggs, and Nuts Group
2–3 Servings

Vegetable Group
3–5 Servings

Fruit Group
2–4 Servings

Bread, Cereal, Rice, and Pasta Group
2–4 Servings

The Food Guide Pyramid

The American Diabetes Association, along with The American Dietetic Association, has written its own dietary guidelines that agree with those of the U.S. government. These guidelines can help you to see that your whole family eats a healthy diet. Your dietitian or other health-care provider can help you to plan meals that are both healthy and enjoyable.

Carbohydrates and sugars

Carbohydrates are found in fruits, vegetables, bread, cereal, milk, rice, potatoes, and pasta. Foods like bread, potatoes, and pasta are called starches or complex carbohydrates. The body breaks them down into glucose. It takes a little more time to break down complex carbohydrates into glucose than carbohydrates that are closer in form to glucose, such as candy, table sugar, and fruit juice

As explained in *What Is Diabetes*, glucose is the body's main energy source. Before it can be used as energy, glucose must get inside the body's cells. Insulin is the key that opens the cell doors, letting the glucose in. People with type I diabetes don't make insulin, so glucose stays in their blood instead of entering the cells.

Sugar. Sugar is a carbohydrate. For many years, health professionals thought that people with diabetes should avoid foods that contain sugar. We now know, however, that foods that contain sugar, when eaten as part of a meal, have about the same effect on blood glucose levels as other carbohydrates. For example, a dessert brownie that has 15 grams of sugar will affect your child's blood glucose level about the same as a dinner potato with margarine, which has about 15 grams of carbohydrate. This means that foods containing sugar can be part of your child's meal plan as long as

♦ they are eaten in small amounts (preferably with a complete meal)
♦ your child's blood glucose levels are checked regularly
♦ you monitor the total amount of carbohydrate in your child's diet

It's a good idea to limit your child's consumption of sugary foods. Most of these foods have little nutritional value and they are often high in fat. Talk to your dietitian about how to fit sugary foods into your child's meal plan.

Fruit and fruit juice. Fruits and fruit juice contain natural sugar, but they also contain fiber and other important nutrients. Your dietitian will recommend how much fruit your child with diabetes should eat at each meal or snack.

Sugary foods usually make blood glucose rise quickly. Complex carbohydrates and protein usually make it rise more slowly and can prevent it from dropping again. That's why it's a good idea to give your child a sandwich or crackers with cheese or peanut butter when her blood glucose is low. (See *Hypoglycemia*, page 63.)

At certain times you may want to give your child fruit juice or a sugary food purposely to raise her blood glucose. The following are examples of times when you may want to do this:

♦ to balance a low blood glucose reading
♦ during or after exercise

♦ during a long gap between meals
♦ on sick days

Fat and cholesterol

Unless your child is younger than 2, her meal plan limits the amount of fat and cholesterol that she eats. The U.S. government's healthy eating guidelines advise all Americans over age 2 to eat less fat (especially saturated fat) and cholesterol to reduce the chances of getting heart disease.

Saturated fat and cholesterol are found mostly in animal products, including butter, lard, whole milk, and fatty meats. Using low-fat milk and cheese and eating lean meat will help you and your child to eat less saturated fat.

HOW DO I DO MEAL PLANNING?

Meal plans generally include three meals and two or three snacks a day. It is a good idea for your child to eat at about the same time most days. Eating at regular times helps to balance the way insulin works in your child's body.

But your child's schedule won't be the same every day. Gym class at school may be changed to a different time. Going out on a family picnic may mean eating lunch later than usual. It's okay to adjust your child's meal plan when your child's or the family's schedule changes. For example, when you know that a meal is going to be eaten later than usual, make sure your child eats a snack to keep her blood glucose from getting too low.

There are many ways to do meal planning for children with diabetes. What's right for your child depends on the kind of foods she likes to eat, as well as on her age, appetite, weight, and activity level. Your health-care provider can help you to find what works best for your child.

What are exchanges?

Exchanges are one way of making meal planning easier for people with diabetes. Your doctor or dietitian can give you a booklet called *Exchange Lists for Meal Planning* that explains how to plan meals using exchanges. This booklet divides foods into lists, including:

♦ starches

- ♦ meats
- ♦ vegetables
- ♦ fruits
- ♦ milk
- ♦ fat

A food on any one of these lists can be exchanged, or traded, for any other food on the same list. Your child's individual meal plan tells you how many portions, or exchanges, can be chosen from each list at a meal. Using exchanges helps to make sure that your child eats the right amounts of nutrients every day.

Planning Meals Using Exchanges

The following are examples of meals you might plan for your child using the Exchange Lists (2,200-calorie plan)

Breakfast: 1 milk, 1 fruit, 2 starches, 2 meats
  1 cup (8 oz.) skim milk (1 milk)
  half-cup (4 oz.) orange juice (1 fruit)
  2 slices of bread (2 starches)
  2 slices of lean ham (2 meats)

Lunch: 3 starches, 2 meats, 1 fruit, 1 milk, 3 fats
  grilled cheese sandwich (2 starches, 2 meats, 1 fat)
  small apple (1 fruit)
  1 cup (8 oz.) skim milk (1 milk)
  1 oz. pretzels (1 starch)

Afternoon snack: 1 starch, 1 milk
  3 cups air-popped popcorn (1 starch)
  1 cup (8 oz.) nonfat yogurt (1 milk)

Dinner: 3 starches, 3 meats, 1 fruit, 1 milk, 2 fats, 2 vegetables
  salad with 1 tbsp. dressing (1 vegetable, 1 fat)
  medium potato (1 starch)
  3 oz. baked chicken (3 meats)
  2" roll (1 starch)
  green beans (1 vegetable)
  baked apple (1 fruit)
  1 cup (8 oz.) skim milk (1 milk)

Bedtime snack: 1 starch, 1 meat, 1 milk
  1/2 turkey sandwich (1 starch, 1 meat)
  1 cup (8 oz.) milk (1 milk)

Carbohydrate counting

Carbohydrate counting is another way of making meal planning easier. To do this, you first add up all the carbohydrates to be eaten for each meal. You then use this number and your child's current blood glucose number to determine the insulin dosage to be given before the meal.

You will need to know how sensitive your child's body is to carbohydrate. This means figuring out how much carbohydrate 1 unit of insulin can take care of. A unit of insulin may cover 20 grams of carbohydrate in one person but less than 10 grams of carbohydrate in another. To find this, your child will need to monitor her blood glucose levels before and after meals, count carbohydrate totals in each meal, and relate them to units of insulin taken before each meal. Then you can figure out about how many units of insulin will cover a certain amount of carbohydrate. This diabetes management tool is for kids and their parents who like math!

This system can work well for people doing intensive diabetes management with either multiple daily injections or an insulin pump. Both of these type of diabetes management are better for older children, over 7 or 8 years old. The dietitian on your health-care team can show you how to get started counting carbohydrates.

Alternative sweeteners

Alternative sweeteners are products that can be used instead of sugar to sweeten food. People with diabetes can safely use alternative sweeteners. Most (but not all) alternative sweeteners have few calories. Four kinds of alternative sweeteners are now available:

- ◆ **Saccharin** is about 400 times as sweet as sugar. It has been used for many years to sweeten many food products. Saccharin can safely be used by people with diabetes. A possible disadvantage of saccharin is that it can leave a slight bitter aftertaste.
- ◆ **Aspartame** is about 200 times as sweet as sugar. Most people, including people with diabetes, can safely use aspartame. However, aspartame is not safe for people who have a rare condition called phenylketonuria (PKU). Aspartame can't be used for cooking because it breaks down when heated.

- ◆ **Acesulfame-K** contains natural flavors extracted from fruits. It can be used safely by people with diabetes or PKU.
- ◆ **Fructose** (fruit sugar) is naturally found in fruit, so it is not calorie-free like other artificial sweeteners. It is a carbohydrate that is broken down by the body more slowly than other sugars. Fructose should be counted as carbohydrate in a meal plan for diabetes. In an exchange diet, it is counted as a fruit exchange.

BECOMING A FOOD DETECTIVE

Foods affect people in different ways. You may begin to notice that some foods affect your child's blood glucose level more than others. For example, eating spaghetti may make blood glucose run higher than eating mashed potatoes and meat loaf. Waffles for breakfast may cause a rise in blood glucose before lunch, but cereal may not. Pizza prepared at different shops may have different effects on blood glucose.

This doesn't mean that your child can't eat certain foods. As you become aware of the effects that different foods have, you can use this knowledge to balance these foods with insulin or exercise.

For example, if you know that crackers make your child's blood glucose run higher than pretzels, you may want to pack crackers for her snack on a day when she is going skating. If waffles make blood glucose run high, you know that your child will need extra insulin on "waffle days."

Keeping a daily log of everything your child eats can help you identify how different foods affect your child's blood glucose. You can use this food diary to adjust your child's insulin dosage depending on what she is eating.

J oanna's glucose always runs high when she eats pizza. So, on days when Joanna's mother knows she is going to be eating pizza, she gives her a bit more insulin than usual to maintain balance.

This sort of detective work takes time and effort to do. The reward is that you and your child have more control over her diabetes. Your dietitian and diabetes educator can help you become skilled at this task.

HOW CAN I HELP MY CHILD TO ACCEPT MEAL PLANNING?

Even though your child's meal plan can be flexible enough to work in a favorite food or dessert, there may be times when you or she chooses not to eat what everyone else is eating. How you decide to do this depends on the situation, the timing of the food, whether you are able to make an adjustment in insulin easily, your child's frame of mind about it, and what her blood glucose level is. For example, if your child's blood glucose level is running high and she really doesn't care that much for the chocolate cake being served, you may decide to go with the usual meal plan that day and skip the cake. Or, if she feels strongly about eating the cake, you may work out a compromise.

As your child grows and learns about diabetes, it will be important that she understands the food groups and how each affects her blood glucose levels. Learning this will take time and patience but it will allow her to make her own decisions about when to choose pretzels over a cupcake.

Many families find that it helps if everyone eats the same meal instead of serving a separate meal for the child with diabetes. That way, there's no reason for the child with diabetes to feel different. Besides, a meal that is healthy for a person with diabetes is healthy for everyone.

Sometimes your child can have food that looks a lot like the food others are eating. For example, when her friends are having fried hamburgers, potato chips, and cola, your child can have a broiled hamburger, pretzels, and a diet soda. Your child's food looks a lot like the friends' food, but it is lower in fat and sugar.

With a bit of planning, your child can have lunch at school with her friends. Many schools give out copies of lunch menus to help parents who need to plan their children's meals ahead of time. Using these menus, you can help your child choose foods that fit in with her meal plan.

Involving your child in planning meals and snacks can be helpful. She may find it easier to follow a meal plan that she has helped to plan.

Some children may go through a phase of hiding candy in their school locker or having a cookie and ice cream binge after school. This kind of behavior may be a protest at "feeling different" or a test to see what will happen. Try not to get upset with your child if this happens. Ask her to let you know if she snacks on sweets because this information will help you in adjusting insulin.

Having a meal plan that is flexible and includes some sweets may prevent your child from bingeing or sneaking food. Try to build a relationship of trust with your child by talking to her openly and by praising her when she follows her meal plan.

Seven-year-old Amy's blood test results were often high when she came home from school. Her parents suspected the problem was caused by eating extra treats on the school bus. Her mother put Amy on her lap, hugged her, and asked her if she was eating candy with her friends. Amy admitted that she was. She said she wanted to join in with what her friends were doing. Amy and her mother talked about how hard it was not for her to eat candy when her friends were eating it. Her mother explained that eating too many candies made Amy's glucose high and that high glucose made Amy feel ill and tired. In the end they decided that Amy should take small boxes of raisins with her to share with her friends on the school bus. She could eat the raisins and feel like "one of the gang." After that, Amy's after-school blood test results improved.

COPING WITH SCHEDULE CHANGES

A schedule change will sometimes prevent your child from following her usual meal plan. If sticking to the meal plan means singling out and upsetting your child, it may be better to adjust the meal plan for the schedule change. However, your child's diabetes control may not be the best on these occasions.

A special event at school may mean that the time of your child's lunch hour or gym class is changed for a few days. If you know about this change ahead of time, you can add a snack to the meal plan or adjust the insulin dose to maintain balance. It can help to talk with your child's teachers and ask them to inform you whenever there is a change to the school schedule that affects your child's meal times or exercise routine, so you can plan ahead. (See *Communicating With Your Child's School and Teachers*, page 88.)

If lunch is delayed for more than an hour for some reason, giving your child any food that contains about 15 grams of carbohydrate (such as 6 low-fat crackers, 2 pretzels, or 3 graham crackers) will prevent low blood glucose. Additional snacks are helpful any time your child gets extra exercise or has to wait longer than usual between meals.

PARTIES AND HOLIDAYS

Many party foods are sweet and high in fat. If your child is going to a party, you may want to get in touch with the hosts beforehand to find out what kind of food is being served. If a lot of high-fat, high-sugar foods are on the menu, you may want to offer to bring some healthier foods.

For example, popcorn or Chex snacks wrapped with colorful bows can be served instead of cupcakes at a child's birthday party. Most parents will welcome the offer.

It's okay for your child to eat birthday cake or other party foods. It's worth some planning ahead to help keep your child from feeling left out. Before your child goes to a party, it's a good idea to make plans with her about how she wants to eat and why. Then you can try some options:

♦ Talk to her about scraping off some of the cake icing to reduce the amount of carbohydrate she eats.
♦ Adjust insulin or alter the amount of food at other meals or the timing of meals to account for the party foods. Sometimes the extra food is substituted for a snack or part of a meal. At other times, it's eaten in addition to the child's usual food.
♦ Plan a calorie-burning family outing after the party.

Your diabetes educator can help you to plan for special events. The chart on page 57 provides some ideas for children's parties that your child with diabetes can enjoy.

Eating is often a central part of holiday celebrations. Usually the food is plentiful and there are lots of special sweet dishes. Having diabetes need not prevent your child from enjoying these special occasions. With careful planning, she can eat most of the same foods that everyone else is eating. The chart on page 58

Healthy Party Ideas For Children With Diabetes

♦ Have a soft-dough pretzel-making party. Children enjoy molding the dough into different shapes and then eating their creations as snacks.
♦ Have a theme party centered on an acceptable food item.
  – At a Peanut Party you can serve fresh peanuts and peanut-butter sandwiches as snacks. Activities can include a peanut hunt and peanut relay races.
  – At an Apple Party children might dunk for apples; decorate apple-people with raisins, toothpicks, and grapes; and enjoy an apple dessert.
  – At a Mexican party, children can put together their own tacos.
  – At a Hawaiian luau, you can serve pineapple and chicken and the children can wear grass skirts and leis.
♦ Take children swimming or on an outing to the zoo. Your library can be a good source of ideas for children's activities that focus on something other than food.
♦ Put candles on a pizza instead of on a cake.

provides some ideas for ways to make holidays both fun and safe for your child with diabetes.

The excitement of holidays can affect children's blood glucose levels. For example, the thrill of opening presents on Christmas morning can distract a child from eating and cause low blood glucose. You can adjust for this by reducing insulin or reminding your child to eat.

EATING OUT

Like other special occasions involving food, eating out can be safe and enjoyable for people with diabetes. Many restaurants and fast food chains can provide information on the calorie and fat content of menu items. Some offer exchange lists to make meal planning easier. Ask questions about things on the menu. Most restaurant staff will be happy to answer your questions.

Eating away from home means food won't always show up when you expect it. If your meal is taking longer to appear on the table than you planned and you're worried about your child's blood glucose dropping low, ask for some rolls (light on butter) or crackers or a soft drink. If you're at an event, such as a wedding reception, where you're not sure when food will be served, think about waiting to inject insulin until you know food is in reach.

Hints For Holidays

Holidays are extra special times for children. The following hints can help your child with diabetes enjoy the festivities.

- **Easter:** Fill an Easter basket with treats other than food, such as coloring books or stickers. Or fill plastic eggs with promises of treats, like a chance to stay up late or a trip to a museum or to the movies.
- **Halloween:** Have your child trade that trick-or-treat bag full of sweets for a present she has been wanting. Or auction it off to the rest of the family for spending money. Instead of trick-or-treating, collect money for a good cause. Or take a trip to visit a haunted house or see a scary movie.
- **Thanksgiving:** Make turkey decorations out of pine cones or a fresh pineapple (the pineapple top is the "tail"). Make a sugar-free pumpkin pie or use skim milk and artificial sweetener instead of cream and sugar. After Thanksgiving dinner, plan a brisk hike through the woods with relatives or friends. This is a good way to lower blood glucose and use up some of the calories from the meal.
- **Christmas or Hanukkah:** Try to serve nonsweet foods. Most guests won't mind because they have lots of other opportunities to eat sweets. They may even appreciate the change of pace.

Helpful Hints For Eating Out

- Ask if food is breaded or fried.
- Request that dishes be broiled rather than fried.
- Ask if sauces are sweetened.
- Request that dishes be served without butter, fats, or oils.
- Ask that salad dressings, margarine, sour cream, and sauces be served "on the side."
- Ask for "lite" or sugar-free syrup, jelly, or dressing.

If you think your child's soft drink isn't sugar free:
Sometimes you may not be sure that the diet soda you ordered is really sugar free. To find out, try dipping a urine test strip into the drink. If the strip turns dark, there is probably sugar in the drink. Most sugar-free soft drinks will not cause the strip to turn dark. But drinks made from sugar-free powdered mixes (such as sugar-free Kool-Aid and iced tea mixes) *will* change the strips because they contain small amounts of substances similar to sugar. You may want to play it safe by ordering a canned drink that you know is sugar-free.

When children first develop diabetes they may wonder, "Can I still play with my friends and do sports?" The answer is definitely yes. Many professional athletes have diabetes, including basketball player Chris Dudley of the Portland Trail Blazers and professional football player Jonathan Hayes of the Pittsburgh Steelers.

All children should be encouraged to be physically active, and children with diabetes are no exception. Regular exercise has many benefits:

♦ It strengthens the heart and lungs.
♦ It builds muscle and improves flexibility in the joints.
♦ It builds confidence and reduces stress.
♦ It provides interaction with other children.

For people with diabetes physical activity has an added benefit: It helps to lower blood glucose levels. When the body's muscles are working, more glucose moves into muscle tissue instead of staying in the blood. Children who begin exercising regularly usually need less insulin than they did before. (But be sure to consult with your doctor before initiating any change in your child's insulin dose.)

Taking part in gym class and team sports also helps your child to develop social skills, make friends, and feel like "one of the gang."

Getting *regular* exercise is important for people with diabetes because of the need to balance the effect of exercise with food and insulin. Activities that meet regularly, like swimming or soccer, make it easier to plan meals and insulin doses.

This chapter provides general guidance on making physical activity and exercise as safe as possible for children with diabetes. If you have specific questions about what's right for your child, check with your doctor or diabetes educator.

BEING PREPARED FOR UNPLANNED GAMES AND ACTIVITIES

Your health-care provider can help you to make regular, planned exercise an enjoyable and safe part of your child's life. But children's lives also involve a lot of unplanned activity. For example, your child may take part in a spontaneous basketball game or some other strenuous activity with friends.

Because exercise lowers blood glucose levels, unplanned physical activity may cause your child's blood glucose to drop. The simplest way to prevent this is to always carry snack foods like crackers with peanut butter or cheese, which contain carbohydrate and protein to boost blood glucose levels. It's a good idea for your child to eat a snack before taking part in any unplanned physical activity.

Depending on how strenuous the activity is, additional snacks may be needed during the play or afterward. These snacks are eaten in addition to the child's usual meals. They replace the glucose that the muscle cells use during exercise.

How much food your child needs to eat depends on what his blood glucose level is and how strenuous the activity is (see **Guidelines for Snacks and Exercise**, this page). Checking blood glucose levels before the activity can help you or your child to decide how much food to eat. (See *Glucose Testing*.)

Guidelines for Snacks and Exercise

The following are general guidelines for snacks before exercise. A dietitian may suggest other guidelines for your child. Consult your health-care provider for specific advice.

Light activities (such as walking, bowling, or ping pong)

Carbohydrate need:	20–30 grams per hour of exercise
Blood glucose 70–180 mg/dl:	3–5 pretzels or 2–3 cups of popcorn would provide 10–15 grams of carbohydrate
Blood glucose over 180 mg/dl:	A snack may not be required before light exercise, or it can be eaten after the exercise.

Vigorous activities (such as jogging or competitive swimming)

Carbohydrate need:	30–60 grams per hour of exercise
Blood glucose 70–180 mg/dl:	1–2 sandwiches or 1 sandwich and 1 fruit eaten before exercise provides enough complex carbohydrate and protein for 1 hour of strenuous exercise.
Blood glucose above 180 mg/dl:	1 sandwich or 1 fruit

WHAT ELSE CAN I DO TO BE SURE MY CHILD CAN ALWAYS PLAY SAFELY?

As well as carrying snack foods like crackers or pretzels, it's a good idea for youngsters to carry a backup source of glucose to guard against "lows." Always keep a package of sugar cubes, hard candy, or glucose tablets in your child's backpack, purse, or pocket.

One athletic youngster keeps a pack of glucose tablets in his football helmet so it's available during a game if he needs it. Some parents buy their child gym shorts and sweat suits with pockets so he can carry sugary snacks.

Talk with your child's gym teachers and sports coaches about the symptoms of low blood glucose and what to do if it occurs (see *Hypoglycemia*, page 63).

Lengthy exercise (like a day-long ski trip) or a major change in routine (like the start of football training) requires special planning. Talk to your health-care provider about how to prepare for these kinds of activities.

It's important that your child exercise with a partner whenever possible in case he has an episode of low blood glucose and needs help.

Strenuous exercise like jogging or swimming laps can affect glucose levels up to 24 hours later. Even if your child snacks before strenuous exercise, he may still have low blood glucose afterward. Some parents find they need to check their child's blood glucose before they go to bed and during the night on a day when the child has had more exercise than usual.

BALANCING EXERCISE AND INSULIN

What if you take all these precautions and your child still has "lows" during gym class or while playing games? If that happens, your child's insulin dosage may need to be decreased.

Insulin may also need to be decreased if your child is taking part in a vigorous sport like swimming, soccer, or football, and doesn't want to "load up" on food beforehand. Big changes in your child's insulin dosage should only be made after discussion with your doctor. You can, however, learn how to fine-tune your child's dosage to control glucose levels. (See *Adjusting Insulin at Home*, page 31.)

Children should not exercise if ketones are present in their urine. Ketones are a sign that the body lacks insulin. Exercise will speed up the loss of insulin and cause more ketones. (See *Urine Testing*, page 41.)

Precautions for Safe Physical Activity

Before exercise:
♦ Check blood glucose level
♦ Eat an extra carbohydrate-rich snack

At all times:
♦ Carry sugar cubes or glucose tablets to treat "lows"
♦ Don't exercise if ketones are present in the urine
♦ During strenuous exercise, stop every 30 minutes to eat or drink a carbohydrate-rich snack
♦ Exercise with a buddy if possible

As a general rule, you can consider your child's diabetes to be reasonably well-controlled if her blood glucose level is within the target range most of the time and she does not get severe symptoms of low blood glucose.

Sometimes, however, the balance of insulin, food, and exercise is upset and your child may show signs of high or low blood glucose. Eating different amounts or different types of food or being more or less active than usual will affect your child's blood glucose levels. Differences in the way the body absorbs insulin or in how hormones in the body respond to insulin may also cause blood glucose levels to get too high or too low.

Most of the time you'll be aware in advance of situations that might cause high or low blood glucose. Sometimes, however, it can happen for no apparent reason. Knowing how to identify high and low blood glucose levels, and what to do when they happen, can help you to act quickly to protect your child's health.

HYPOGLYCEMIA (LOW BLOOD GLUCOSE)

Hypoglycemia is the most common problem in children with diabetes. Most of the time it is mild and can be easily treated by giving the child a sweet food.

Food raises blood glucose levels and insulin and exercise lower them. Low blood glucose can occur when the balance of insulin, food, and exercise is upset. The body can't control insulin that's given as an injection in the same way it controls insulin that the body makes itself. Once an injection is given, the insulin can't be stopped or slowed down. So if too much insulin is available, blood glucose levels will drop too low.

People with diabetes have to control their own blood glucose levels because their bodies don't do it for them. Eating meals and getting insulin injections at regular times and snacking before exercise help to prevent glucose levels from getting too low.

Hypoglycemia needs to be treated promptly to prevent blood glucose levels from getting so low that the brain is deprived of glucose. Too little glucose in the brain can cause severe symptoms, such as:

♦ sleepiness and unresponsiveness
♦ seizures
♦ unconsciousness

How can I tell if my child's blood glucose is low?

The symptoms of low blood glucose may be different each time it happens. Sometimes your child may have no obvious symptoms. For these reasons, it is a good idea to teach a child with diabetes to tell you whenever she feels "strange" in any way.

In children under 3, misbehavior or crankiness may be a sign that the child's blood glucose is low. Very young children can't tell you when they're not feeling well, so you need to be on the lookout for warning signs. Frequent blood glucose tests can help to relieve parental anxiety.

Most parents learn to recognize the symptoms of low blood glucose in their child. It is a good idea to talk with your child's teachers (and other adults whom your child has contact with) about the symptoms of low blood glucose.

A quick-witted teacher reported this experience with a usually pleasant and calm student: While waiting in the cafeteria line at lunch, the youngster became irritable and punched a classmate for no reason. The teacher guessed that the cause of the behavior might be low blood glucose and gave the student a glass of orange juice and some crackers. In about 15 minutes, after the juice and crackers began to raise her blood glucose level, the student became her usual pleasant self again.

Scientists think that low blood glucose may continue to affect a child's learning ability for a while (perhaps an hour or so) after it has been treated. A period when your child's glucose level is low may not be the best time for her to take an important exam or give a presentation. This is another reason why it's a good idea to talk to your child's teachers about low blood glucose.

Sometimes your child may feel nervous, anxious, or tired and think it's because of low blood glucose. She may have some of the symptoms of low blood glucose if her glucose level drops quickly from high to normal. The best thing to do if you or your child suspect that blood glucose is low is to do a blood test.

If the child has symptoms of low blood glucose but the blood test shows that glucose isn't low, she may be experiencing a fast drop in blood glucose without being in any danger of hypoglycemia. Giving her a few crackers to eat will help the "low" feelings subside. In a few minutes she can return to her normal activities. If blood glucose levels are not low, eating a carbohydrate snack is not urgent.

If in doubt, treat. If you think your child may have low blood glucose but you can't do a blood test right away, give the child something sweet to eat. The treatment will not do any harm even if the child's glucose level is not low.

Preventing low blood glucose

Low blood glucose can usually be prevented by:
- ◆ testing glucose levels regularly
- ◆ following the recommended meal plan
- ◆ making sure the insulin dose is correct
- ◆ eating extra snacks before exercise that is unplanned or more strenuous than usual

You may need to remind your child that testing blood glucose helps to make sure that the insulin dose and meal plan are right.

If your child follows these guidelines and still has frequent episodes of low blood glucose, talk to your doctor or diabetes educator. Your child's insulin dose or meal plan may need to be changed.

If you and your child are trying to keep her glucose levels near normal, you can expect that she will have mild episodes of low blood glucose occasionally. While not desirable, they are probably not dangerous and are easily treated.

Treating low blood glucose—mild to moderate symptoms

Low blood glucose needs to be treated quickly. The way to treat it is to give the child a sweet food like fruit juice, raisins, or glucose tablets, followed by four crackers. A candy bar is not the best choice because it is high in fat and calories. But if a candy bar is the only food available, it is an acceptable treatment for low blood glucose.

Depending on how much food is already in the child's stomach, it may take 10 to 20 minutes for the blood glucose level to rise. If your child isn't feeling better in 20 minutes, check her blood glucose level again. If it's still low, repeat the treatment.

A low blood glucose episode may occur just before a snack or a meal. If this happens, give the child something sweet and see that she eats the snack or meal as soon as possible.

If a snack or meal isn't coming up soon, give the child a snack food containing complex carbohydrate and protein to follow the sweet food. Crackers with cheese or peanut butter, cereal and milk, or half a sandwich are good choices. This food is eaten in addition to the day's usual meals.

> David was going on a long hike with a group of children. His mother told the counselor in charge to give David something sweet if he showed symptoms of low blood glucose. When David felt shaky at the beginning of the hike, the counselor gave him sugar cubes. Twenty minutes later David felt shaky again. The counselor gave him more sugar cubes. This happened every 20 minutes during the trip. To prevent these later episodes the counselor could have given David a complex carbohydrate and protein (such as a cheese or peanut butter sandwich) at the beginning of the hike.

Treating low blood glucose—severe symptoms

A child who is very drowsy, unconscious, or unable to eat, drink, or swallow may be experiencing severe low blood glucose.

Do *not* put anything in the child's mouth if she is unconscious or likely to choke or clamp down on your fingers. If the child can't or won't swallow, you will need to give her an injection of **glucagon** to raise blood glucose levels. (Glucagon is a hormone normally made by the pancreas. Your doctor can give you a prescription for it.)

The injection usually takes effect in 15 to 20 minutes. If the child does not respond within that time, contact your doctor or take the child to an emergency room right away.

Treating Low Blood Glucose

Mild to moderate symptoms *(child is alert and can swallow):*

Treat right away with a sweet food:
1/2–3/4 cup orange or apple juice
1–2 glucose tablets or doses of glucose gel
2–4 LifeSavers (or similar product)
5 small gumdrops
1–2 tbsp. honey
6 oz. nondiet soda
2 tbsp. cake icing (such as Cake Mate tube icing)

Follow a few minutes later with:
2–4 soda crackers and 1 oz. of cheese
OR 1 tbsp. peanut butter (or other "complex" carbohydrate and protein)

Don't overtreat: 1/2 cup (4 oz.) of orange juice or a glucose drink, followed by 4 crackers, should be enough to relieve symptoms. Remember that sugar takes time to be absorbed. Give more sugar after about 15 minutes if the symptoms don't go away.

Severe symptoms *(child is very sleepy, very shaky, unconscious, or unable to eat, drink, or swallow):*

Treat *immediately* with an injection of glucagon. The standard dose is 1 mg. However, children up to age 6 usually only need 0.5 mg (half the standard dose). The injection should take effect in 15–20 minutes. If the child doesn't respond, call your doctor or take the child to an emergency room.

Being prepared for low blood glucose emergencies

It's a good idea for everyone who takes insulin to always carry something sweet for emergencies. Packages of glucose tablets, sugar cubes, or hard candy are useful because they are easy to carry. It's also a good idea to carry a sandwich, cheese or peanut butter crackers, or some other food containing complex carbohydrate and protein.

You should keep a glucagon kit at home and in a travel kit for use in an episode of severe low blood glucose. Your doctor or nurse can show you how to use the kit. Be sure that babysitters and others who take care of your child know how to use it, too.

Adults caring for a child with diabetes often are afraid to treat symptoms of low blood glucose because they think that eating sweets will harm the child. Be sure that your child's teachers, coaches, babysitters, and so on know what the symptoms of low blood glucose are and that sugar is the proper treatment.

> **Remember**: Check blood glucose if you're not sure whether your child is "low." But if you can't test, treat with something sweet.

Should my child wear a medical ID tag?

It's a good idea for everyone who has diabetes, including young children, to wear a medical identification tag at all times. These tags can save lives in an emergency.

The kind of tag you choose will depend on your child's age and preference. It is most important that the tag be in a style your child will wear. For young children, ankle chains are probably the best choice. Neck chains are not suitable for infants and preschoolers, who are likely to play with the chains and may break them or choke on them.

A variety of colorful nylon bracelets are available for children. Teenagers may prefer a necklace-style chain. Sewing ID tags into the child's undershirts is another option.

Makers and styles of medical ID tags change frequently. Ask your diabetes educator or pharmacist for a current list of suppliers or see the *Buyers Guide to Diabetes Supplies*, published every October in *Diabetes Forecast*, the monthly magazine of the American Diabetes Association.

You may want to carry a wallet card at all times with your child's medical information on it. You can get wallet cards in most pharmacies and from American Diabetes Association chapters or affiliates.

HYPERGLYCEMIA (HIGH BLOOD GLUCOSE)

Blood glucose levels can rise when the body gets too little insulin or too much food, or when the child is less active than usual. Physical and emotional stress can also cause blood glucose levels to rise. Having a cold or sore throat, getting braces, worrying about exams, or going through the hormonal changes of puberty may all cause hyperglycemia.

Preventing and treating hyperglycemia

The best way to prevent hyperglycemia is to test blood glucose levels regularly to detect high blood glucose (see *The Nitty-Gritty 2—Glucose Testing*). This will enable you to adjust your child's insulin dose, food intake, or exercise level to prevent symptoms from occurring. Taking insulin regularly and following the recommended meal plan are also important in preventing hyperglycemia.

Unless a child is overweight and trying to shed pounds, it's not a good idea to cut down on food to lower glucose levels. Your child needs food to grow and develop normally. Her meal plan is designed to give her the nutrients she needs. Spacing meals and snacks farther apart may help if your child often gets high blood glucose, but talk this over with your doctor or diabetes educator before trying it.

KETOACIDOSIS AND DIABETIC COMA

Ketones are acid waste products that are created when the body burns fat to get the energy it needs. They build up in the blood and spill into the urine. Very high levels of ketones in the blood and urine is called **ketoacidosis.**

Diabetic coma can be a result of severe or prolonged ketoacidosis. A person can have ketoacidosis without being in a coma. Untreated, ketoacidosis is life-threatening.

If your child is receiving enough insulin for her needs, she will not get ketoacidosis even if her blood glucose level is high. Eating too much at dinner one night will not cause ketoacidosis if the body has enough insulin to meet its needs.

However, ketoacidosis may occur if the child has very high blood glucose and is vomiting. This is because the body makes larger amounts of hormones like adrenaline when your child is sick. These hormones help the body fight illness but they also block the action of insulin. This is why you *always* give your child insulin when she is sick—even if she is eating less than usual.

Preventing and treating ketoacidosis

You can prevent ketoacidosis by checking urine for ketones daily and by treating illness and hyperglycemia promptly with your doctor's assistance.

Ketoacidosis must be treated promptly. Call your doctor right away if your child has any of the problems listed in the chart below.

Ketoacidosis usually needs to be treated with an infusion of intravenous fluids. It may be treated in the emergency room, or a short hospital stay may be necessary.

When to Call the Doctor Immediately

Check with your child's doctor to learn when you should call. *Always call right away if your child has any of the following problems. Your child may be developing ketoacidosis.*
- Moderate levels of ketones in the urine (see *Urine Testing*, page 41.)
- Ketones in the urine for more than one urine test
- Dehydration (symptoms include: sunken eyes; dry, cracked lips; dry mouth; skin remains "pinched up" after it is pinched)
- Persistent vomiting*
- Any change in alertness; drowsiness, labored breathing
- Fruity-smelling breath (like fruity chewing gum or nail polish remover)
- Abdominal pain

If you can't reach the doctor, take the child to an emergency room right away.

* Vomiting can be caused by many illnesses. It is always a potentially serious problem and can cause ketoacidosis.

REBOUND (SOMOGYI EFFECT)

Rebound is an abnormal increase in blood glucose that occurs after an episode of low blood glucose. It is called the Somogyi effect after the doctor who first identified it, Michael Somogyi.

When blood glucose levels fall below normal, the body usually responds by producing extra adrenaline, glucagon, and other hormones that help the body deal with stress. These hormones cause the liver to store glucose and release it into the blood.

This process can help to prevent your child's blood glucose level from dropping too low. Sometimes, however, the adrenaline and glucagon can go on working for hours after blood glucose levels are back to normal. This can cause high blood glucose several hours after an episode of low blood glucose.

One clue that your child may have rebound is a pattern of blood glucose tests that read low, high, low, high, etc. Small amounts of ketones in the urine may be another clue. If your child has wide swings in blood glucose levels over the course of a few days, it's a good idea to talk to your doctor or diabetes educator.

Rebound is often treated by reducing the insulin dose. But it's not a good idea to treat rebound on your own. Seek help from your doctor.

DAWN PHENOMENON

People with diabetes frequently experience a rise in blood glucose levels very early in the morning. This increase is called the *dawn phenomenon* because it occurs at around 5 a.m. and because no one knows for sure *why* it happens.

Some scientists think that the dawn phenomenon may occur because the insulin that was injected the night before is all used up. The dawn phenomenon can be prevented by increasing the evening insulin dose or by giving the evening insulin dose at bedtime.

Talk to your doctor if you notice that your child has high blood glucose levels very early in the morning.

HOW TO HANDLE SICK DAYS

Children with diabetes do not usually get sick more often than other children. However, children with diabetes need special care when they get colds, the flu, and other illnesses.

It may be helpful for you and your child's doctors to work out in advance a plan for handling sick days. The plan should include:
♦ phone numbers for reaching a doctor at all times
♦ guidelines for when it is important to call
♦ guidelines for adjusting insulin
♦ guidelines for checking blood glucose and adjusting your child's meal plan

Giving insulin during illness

Your child should *always* take insulin–even if she is not eating well. Illness and stress can cause the body to need more insulin.

Children may need higher doses of rapid-acting insulin on sick days to lower blood glucose quickly.

However, if your child is eating poorly or vomiting, she may need less than the usual amount of intermediate-acting insulin. If your child is vomiting or not eating, call your health-care provider right away for advice on adjusting her insulin dose.

Blood and urine testing

It's very important to check blood glucose levels and test urine for ketones more often than usual when your child is sick. The extra tests will help you and the doctor decide how much extra insulin your child needs.

Test blood glucose at least four times a day, and test urine for ketones frequently (several times a day). If your child is vomiting or has large amounts of ketones in the urine, you may need to test both blood and urine every two hours. This stepped-up testing schedule should continue until ketones clear, blood glucose is back to normal, and the child feels better.

Eating during illness

Try to keep your child on her regular meal plan as much as possible. She still needs food to balance insulin. If your child has trouble eating regular foods, try some of the foods in the chart on page 74 (*Easy Foods for Sick Days*). Small meals and extra snacks may be better than three big meals.

Encourage your child to drink lots of fluids, especially if she has a fever. It's very easy for a child to become dehydrated during illness. Dehydration robs the body of needed water and nutrients, can disrupt control of diabetes, and may contribute to ketoacidosis.

If your child is eating, it's a good idea for her to drink water or sugar-free sodas, powdered drink mixes, or iced tea (which have no calories). If your child is *not* eating, is vomiting, has diarrhea, or has ketones in the urine, she needs fluids that contain carbohydrates and calories. Regular cola or ginger ale, gelatin water, popsicles, apple juice, powdered drink mixes, or Pedialyte are good choices.

INFECTIONS

If your child's glucose levels are in her target range, she should not get more infections than other children. However, if she has

Helpful Hints for Sick Days

Your doctor can give you guidance tailor-made for your child, but the following general hints may be helpful.

◆ Reaching the doctor
  Write down phone numbers where you can reach a doctor at all times. Keep these numbers handy.
◆ Insulin
  Your child needs insulin every day and may need extra doses on sick days.
◆ Blood and urine testing
  Check blood glucose levels at least four times a day. Test urine for ketones frequently. If child is vomiting or has large amounts of ketones in the urine, test both blood and urine every two hours.
◆ Meals
  Try small meals and extra snacks. If your child has trouble eating, try special foods (see *Easy Foods for Sick Days* chart). Give child plenty of fluids to drink.
  – *If child is eating*, give sugar-free fluids (such as sugar-free sodas or powdered drink mixes).
  – *If child is not eating*, give fluids that contain sugar and other nutrients (such as nondiet cola, gelatin water (gelatin before it hardens), popsicles, clear broth, Gatorade, or Pedialyte).

frequent high blood glucose, she may be more likely to get infections. This is because bacteria grow well in glucose, and bacteria-fighting cells do not work as well in a high-glucose environment. When glucose is high, it's easier to pick up an infection and harder to shake it off.

Yeast infections

Girls with diabetes may get vaginal infections, especially if they have frequent high blood glucose levels. The most common vaginal infection, often called a "yeast infection," is caused by a fungus called *Candida albicans*.

This fungus is normally present in the skin, mouth, intestinal tract, and vagina. When it multiplies abnormally, it can cause an infection. Having a high level of glucose in the blood and taking some kinds of antibiotics can cause an overgrowth of the fungus.

Symptoms of *Candida* infection include itching, burning, and a thick, white or yellow vaginal discharge that can look like

Easy Foods for Sick Days

These foods are well tolerated by most sick people. They may be also be good substitutes when your child has an upset stomach or has trouble eating regular meals (for example, after getting braces).

Fruit Exchange replacements (10 grams of carbohydrate)
1/2 cup (4 oz.) regular soft drink with sugar (ginger ale or cola)
1/2 cup (4 oz.) fruit juice (orange, grape)
1/2 twin-bar popsicle
1 fruit exchange (1 orange)
2 tbsp. corn syrup or honey
1/4 cup (2 oz.) sweetened gelatin
6 LifeSavers
2 tbsp. (1 oz.) Coke syrup

Starch Exchange replacements (15 grams of carbohydrate)
1/2 cup (4 oz.) ice cream
1/2 cup (4 oz.) cooked cereal
1/4 cup (2 oz.) sherbet
1/2 cup sweetened gelatin
2 cups broth-based soup, reconstituted with water
1 cup cream soup
3/4 cup (6 oz.) regular soft drink with sugar (ginger ale or cola)
1/4 cup (2 oz.) milk shake
1 slice toast
6 soda crackers

Milk Exchange replacements (12 grams of carbohydrate)
5 oz. regular soft drink with sugar (ginger ale or cola)
1 cup eggnog
1 cup (8 oz.) milk

cottage cheese. These infections can usually be treated with over-the-counter suppositories or creams. Improving diabetes control can prevent *Candida* infections. Other ways girls with diabetes can protect themselves from *Candida* infections include:

- ◆ Drying the outside vaginal area thoroughly after a shower, bath, or swim. Yeast is less likely to grow in a dry area.
- ◆ Changing out of a wet bathing suit or other wet clothes quickly.
- ◆ Wearing cotton underwear.
- ◆ Wiping from front to back (away from the vagina) after urination or a bowel movement.

♦ Avoiding wearing nylon (nonbreathing) clothing, such as spandex tights or shorts, for long periods of time.

♦ Avoiding wearing tight jeans if you are prone to infections.

TAKING CARE OF TEETH AND GUMS

Children with diabetes usually do not have more dental problems than other children. They probably eat less candy and sugar than other children, so they should have a lower risk of cavities.

However, **gingivitis** (inflammation of the gums) can be a long-term complication of diabetes. Gingivitis can lead to **periodontitis**, a more severe gum disease in which bone is lost and spaces develop between the gums and the teeth. Following healthy dental practices in childhood may prevent dental problems later on.

It's a good idea to brush teeth twice a day and preferable to do it after every meal. If you treat low blood glucose with sweets at night, try to have your child brush her teeth afterward, or try to wash the sweet food down with water to rinse away sugar between the teeth. Take your child for regular dental checkups. If your child has red, swollen gums or any other dental problem, call your dentist immediately.

If your child needs to have dental surgery, ask your dentist to call your doctor so that the child's insulin dose can be adjusted on the day of surgery and for a few days afterward. If your child's eating habits change after having dental surgery or getting braces, insulin will need to be adjusted. Stay in touch with your doctor or diabetes educator when your child is having dental work done.

THYROID DISEASE

The thyroid is a gland located in the neck. Hormones made by the thyroid gland help to control the way the body works (the **metabolism**).

In *What Is Diabetes* we described how the body can sometimes attack and destroy the cells that make insulin. This is called an **autoimmune** attack. Other antibodies can attack and destroy the thyroid gland, causing thyroid disease. The reasons why autoimmune attacks occur are not known.

When you already have one autoimmune disease (diabetes), you are at increased risk of getting another one. This is why people with diabetes are more likely than other people to get thyroid disease.

There are two kinds of thyroid disease. **Hyperthyroidism** occurs when the thyroid gland makes too much of a hormone called thyroxine. This disease is uncommon in children with diabetes. **Hypothyroidism** occurs when the thyroid does not make enough thyroxine. This disease is more common in children with diabetes than in other children.

When the thyroid gland is damaged by an autoimmune attack, it may get bigger and try to go on making normal amounts of thyroxine. This can cause a swelling in the front part of the neck called a **goiter**. In time, the thyroid can no longer make normal amounts of thyroxine and symptoms of hypothyroidism may appear. These symptoms include:

♦ weight gain
♦ feeling tired or cold
♦ dry skin
♦ hair loss
♦ bowel trouble
♦ irregular menstrual periods

If hypothyroidism is not treated it can affect a child's growth. Your child's doctor can check for hypothyroidism by feeling her thyroid gland and checking the level of thyroxine in the blood. Thyroid disease is easily treated with a pill containing thyroxine, the hormone that the thyroid gland is no longer making.

COMPLICATIONS OF DIABETES

People who have diabetes for a long time may get other diseases that are caused by diabetes. These other diseases are called complications of diabetes. It is rare for children to get these complications. However, your child may be at risk for complications when she has had diabetes for 15 years or more.

Complications of diabetes can include blood vessel problems that lead to kidney disease, heart disease, eye disease, and nerve disease.

In the Diabetes Control and Complications Trial (DCCT), doctors found that maintaining near-normal blood glucose levels ("tight control") prevented or postponed many complications of diabetes. (See *New Thinking About Treating Children With Diabetes*, page 9.)

Achieving tight control takes time, money, and energy. But the DCCT results demonstrate that the effort involved is worthwhile and give people with diabetes more hope for a healthy future.

Although complications of diabetes are rare in childhood, teaching your child healthy habits while she is young can help to prevent or reduce complications when she becomes an adult. For example, learning to keep feet clean when they are bruised or cut will be important later in life to reduce the risk of foot problems.

When your child is 12 years old and has had diabetes for 5 years, she should start seeing an **eye doctor** once a year. If eye disease is found, make sure that she sees an **ophthalmologist** (a doctor who specializes in treating eye diseases), not an **optometrist** (who examines eyes but is not a medical doctor).

Complications and how to prevent them should be discussed in a nonthreatening way with older children and adolescents. Trying to frighten youngsters into changing their behavior by warning them about the risk of complications in the future can have effects that are the opposite of what was intended.

Seventeen-year-old Susan had always had difficulty keeping her blood glucose in the target range. She had trouble following her meal plan and preferred computer games to exercise. A well-meaning uncle thought the best way to motivate Susan was to scare her. "Susan, you'll go blind like your grandmother who had diabetes," he told her. But instead of improving her diabetes care in response to this threat, Susan decided that if she was going to go blind there was no point in making an effort to maintain good glucose control. A better approach would have been to talk with Susan openly about her problems with diabetes care, give her positive encouragement to change, and support her efforts.

If your child is worried about getting complications in the future, it may help to have a talk with her doctor. Your child may also benefit from counseling to help her adjust to living with diabetes. Open discussion of fears can help to make them easier to bear.

As the parent of a child with diabetes, you too may have fears about the future. Feel free to discuss these fears with your health-care provider. Your health-care provider may be able to recommend a counselor who can help you to deal with these worries. Seeking help from a counselor is never a sign of weakness. On the contrary, it's a sign that you want to make life with diabetes the best it can be.

As Your Child Grows Up

Growing up brings special challenges and rewards for both children and parents. Growing up with diabetes is an additional challenge, and growing up healthy brings special rewards, not only for your child but also for you.

All parents worry about their children, but it's natural for you to worry a little more about your child with diabetes. By presenting an overview of situations you may encounter as your child grows up, this chapter may help you to worry a bit less.

WHEN BABY HAS DIABETES

With good medical care, babies with diabetes grow and develop into healthy, active children. Your doctor and other health-care providers can help you to adjust insulin and diet so your infant will grow and gain weight normally. You can expect your baby to roll over, sit up, crawl, and talk at a normal pace.

If your baby is hospitalized, you may find that he briefly loses some of the skills he had developed or goes back to acting the way he did at a younger age. For example, an infant who drank from a cup may insist on a bottle for a while after coming home from the hospital.

This behavior is not caused by diabetes. Any child who undergoes a stressful experience like being hospitalized may cope by seeking comfort in familiar things like a pacifier. Once your baby settles down at home again, he will soon regain any lost skills and continue to develop normally.

How can I tell if my baby has low blood glucose?

Parents are usually most worried about low blood glucose in infancy because babies can't tell their parents that they feel "strange." You will need to learn to look for signs like these that tell you your baby's glucose is low:

♦ sweating
♦ pale skin
♦ irritability

- ◆ tiredness
- ◆ shaking
- ◆ crying
- ◆ enlarged pupils
- ◆ restlessness at night
- ◆ bluish color around the lips

Regular blood glucose tests are very important in babies. Your doctor or nurse educator can help you learn to do these tests. Blood may be taken from heels, toes, or earlobes if little fingers become tender from many fingersticks. See below for a way to test a baby's wet diaper for urine glucose.

It is always a good idea to treat your baby if you are unsure whether he is having a "low." **When in doubt, treat**. (See *Treating a Baby for Low Blood Glucose*, this page.)

Testing a Wet Diaper for Urine Glucose

1. Many brands of disposable diapers contain silica gel to retain moisture and keep baby dry (call the manufacturer to find out). If the diapers you use contain silica gel, place a diaper liner inside your baby's diaper.
2. Pull some of the wet stuffing out of the diaper liner and push it into an empty syringe.
3. Push in the syringe plunger to squeeze out a drop of urine.
4. Place the drop of urine on a test strip and "read" the strip.

Treating a Baby for Low Blood Glucose

1. Give the baby a sugary drink (such as apple juice, sugar water, sugar-sweetened Kool-Aid, or glucose gel). This should have an effect within 20 minutes.
2. Follow with formula or milk (which provides complex carbohydrate and protein). If the baby is eating solids, you may give cereal, vegetables, or meat instead of milk.
3. If the baby won't eat or if symptoms don't improve, give a glucagon injection and **call your doctor**. Make sure you already have instructions from your doctor on how much glucagon to give your baby. Half the usual dose of glucagon (0.5 mg) is often suggested for infants.

Illnesses in infancy

Infants with diabetes don't get infections, colds, or diarrhea more than other babies. If your baby with diabetes does get sick, be sure to follow your doctor's sick-day guidelines.

Sick-day guidelines for babies are the same as for older children (see *How to Handle Sick Days*, page 71). However, a baby can become very sick more quickly than an older child because an infant becomes dehydrated faster. Symptoms of dehydration include:

♦ sunken eyes
♦ dry, cracked lips
♦ dry mouth
♦ skin that remains "pinched up" after being pinched.

Because of the risk of dehydration, make sure your baby continues to take in fluids when he is sick and call your doctor immediately. It's very important to check for ketones frequently when your baby is sick.

Babies with diabetes who have diarrhea should be treated in the same way that any other child with diarrhea would be treated. Usually clear liquids and a "BRAT" diet (Bananas, Rice, Applesauce, dry Toast) are recommended.

Your baby may need less insulin when he has diarrhea or another illness that causes him to eat less than usual. Talk to your doctor or diabetes educator about how to adjust insulin during illness.

If Your Baby Is Vomiting or Has Diarrhea

1. **Call the doctor right away**.
2. Begin to give the baby small amounts of sugary fluids, such as sugar-sweetened Kool-Aid, gelatin water (gelatin before it hardens), or Pedialyte.

If your baby won't eat

All babies go through stages when they won't eat. However, babies with diabetes need food to balance insulin. If your baby won't eat, and isn't yet on solid food, you can try offering other fluids (like juice, sugared water, or Pedialyte). If the baby is on solids, try offering a different food, or else try fluids.

If your baby refuses both solids and fluids, wait 10 minutes and try again. Offering small amounts frequently may be helpful. It's never a good idea to force your infant to eat. You may have to settle for feeding the baby any foods (or fluids) that he likes, such as ice cream, pudding, tapioca, or cookies. For a baby with diabetes, this is always preferable to no food.

Coping with a baby with diabetes

Caring for an infant with diabetes can be difficult and stressful. It's natural for parents to worry about their baby having low blood glucose or not eating or about giving the baby insulin injections.

For your own mental well-being, it's important that you be able to take a break from caring for your child with diabetes for an afternoon, an evening, or a weekend. If you and your spouse are sharing the care, you need uninterrupted time together.

Find a person you trust—for example, a friend, an aunt, a grandparent, or a kindly neighbor—who can care for your baby while you take a break. This caregiver will need general training in diabetes care and an understanding of your baby's care routine.

Some parents find it helps their peace of mind to use a pager or "beeper" when they are away, so that the caregiver can keep in touch with them.

Your doctor, dietitian, diabetes educator, or social worker may be able to suggest additional sources of support when you become very worried or stressed. Asking for help is never a sign of weakness. You have a lot to do and cope with. (See *Asking for Help*, page 109.)

THE PRESCHOOLER WITH DIABETES

Parents of the preschooler with diabetes may have the same feelings of anxiety and helplessness that parents of infants have.

Low blood glucose can still be a big worry. You still need to be on the lookout for signs of low blood glucose (see pages 7 and 64–65) because your child can't always tell you how he is feeling. Frequent blood glucose checks are a good way to reassure yourself that your child is all right.

How can I help my child to accept fingersticks and insulin injections?

Insulin injections and regular blood glucose tests are very important to your child's diabetes care. But the needles and fingersticks can be frightening to a preschooler. The invasion of his body may be especially threatening to a child at this age.

It may help to say to your child: "Yes, I know it hurts" and "You're being very brave." Let the child choose which finger to use for the fingerstick or where to give the insulin injection. Feeling that he has some control over the situation may help to ease the child's anxiety. A Band-Aid to cover the wound and a hug or a kiss when it's over may be all it takes to smooth things out.

You may want to try using stickers or star charts as incentives to help your child accept fingersticks and injections. Explain that every time he has a fingerstick or an injection, he will earn a star or sticker. When he has 20 or 25 stars, he can plan a special treat like a trip to the zoo or the library.

Young children may try to delay fingersticks and injections. They'll say, "Wait just one more minute and I'll be ready." But one minute soon becomes 15 and the child is late for nursery school.

One solution to this problem is to use a cooking timer. Set the timer for 10 minutes and explain that if the child has the fingerstick or injection before the bell rings, he will earn a star. But if the procedure isn't done when the bell rings, he won't get a reward.

Praise your child for being brave and holding still while you give the injection. Try not to scold him for moving during the fingerstick or for being late for an injection.

At times, however, even praise and the offer of rewards may not help. Your child just won't cooperate. Preschoolers may find it hard to understand why they need injections, especially if they don't feel sick.

If this happens, you may have to hold the child or get someone to help you give the injection. This is never pleasant, but your child needs to get insulin regularly. Afterward, it may be helpful to hug your child and explain that you have to give the injections "to keep you well."

Children often express their frustrations and worries through play. Having the preschooler give an injection to a favorite doll or stuffed animal may help the child express his fears.

F our-year-old Larry was terrified of getting his insulin injections. His mother reported that he avoided going to bed at night because he associated waking up in the morning with getting an injection. He woke up during the night with nightmares about the injection. Every morning his parents chased him through the house to give him his insulin.

One day, Larry's mother began including his favorite stuffed animal in the procedure. Before giving Larry his insulin, she went through the entire routine with the toy, including placing a Band-Aid over the injection site. Finally, Larry began giving his "diabetic bunny" the injection. Through play, he was able to express feelings that he couldn't express in words. Eventually, he got over his fear of injections.

How can I get my child to eat regularly?

Getting a youngster with diabetes to eat properly can be just as challenging as giving fingersticks and insulin injections. Young children often try to control and manipulate their parents at meal times.

The most effective way of handling a child who fusses at meals may be to not make an issue of eating or not eating. If the child rejects a meal, offer something else. If that's rejected, try offering orange juice or a piece of fruit. The meal can be offered again later. Watch carefully for signs of low blood glucose if your child is going through a fussy eating phase.

Don't let your child prolong meals so that breakfast, snack, and lunch all seem to run together. Allow a certain amount of time for meals. When the time is up, the meal is over. Without this kind of discipline, your child will be nibbling constantly and his blood glucose will always be out of control.

When your child is not eating well, try not to nag or physically force him to eat. Usually, this kind of pressure will only increase the child's resistance. Instead, try providing positive rewards for behavior you want to encourage. Sometimes when children are not in the mood for eating the entire meal, they may be willing to drink. A carbohydrate-containing beverage, such as milk or flavored milk, may help prevent low blood glucose later on.

It's common for children to want to eat nothing but peanut butter sandwiches for days on end and then to suddenly switch to wanting nothing but hot dogs. As long as the current "fad" food is low in fat and sugar, it's okay to let your child eat as much of it as he wants.

Two-year-old Laura was the youngest of 3 children. School mornings for the family were hectic. Laura got her insulin injection and her breakfast while her mother was busy getting the older children ready for the school bus. Although Laura liked her breakfast cereal, she never finished eating it. Because she had not eaten enough food, Laura always had low blood glucose before lunch. After talking with the diabetes educator about this, Laura's mother changed the family's morning routine. Now she waits until the older children have left for school before giving Laura her insulin injection. Then she makes sure that Laura eats her breakfast and has a midmorning snack to prevent low blood glucose.

What if my child needs to be hospitalized?

Being hospitalized for newly diagnosed diabetes can be very stressful for a youngster. It can be scary and confusing. The child may think that having diabetes or being in the hospital is a punishment for being bad. It's important to try to reassure the youngster that none of these things is his fault.

Your child may be anxious or afraid about being away from home. It helps if you can stay with your child while he is in the hospital. Most children's units will let parents stay with their children.

If you can't stay, it's important to try to tell your child why. Be honest about when you will be back. Leaving the child's favorite toy or blanket can help to ease his anxiety. Pictures or a parent's possession (like a scarf or a handkerchief) are another good reminder of home and family.

For many parents, the period of their child's hospitalization is a time to learn (in a safe environment) as much as they can about their new responsibilities as the parents of a child with diabetes. If your child is not hospitalized when he is diagnosed, you may be able to attend an outpatient program about diabetes care for parents. In either case, diabetes educators will provide help and advice as you learn to give insulin injections and do blood tests.

THE SCHOOL-AGE YEARS

Children ages 6 to 12 usually have a lot of energy and are eager to learn and do things. They have a vivid imagination, a conscience, and the ability to share and cooperate. They display their energy in horseplay, teasing, schoolwork, games, and fantasy. They have an increasing desire for independence, but they still want their parents' protection and authority.

Starting school or moving on to middle school is a new challenge that may cause a child with diabetes to feel insecure at times. He is meeting a lot of new people and facing new demands such as homework and school sports. He may become anxious because his parents aren't always with him.

Parents, in turn, may try to overprotect a child with diabetes. When the child starts going to school, it may be the first time the parent has been separated from the child.

For these reasons, it may be hard for a child with diabetes to be as independent as other children his age. Balancing a child's needs for independence and protection is hard. Yet you help your child most by encouraging him to lead as normal a life as possible while still taking care of his diabetes.

If you have concerns about how to balance your child's needs for independence and protection, you may want to discuss your feelings with your doctor or diabetes educator. School-age children are often ready to do more of their diabetes care than their parents think they can handle. However, they generally feel more secure when a parent or another adult, such as the school nurse or a teacher, supervises and supports their care efforts.

How to handle troublesome periods

As children begin to develop their own identities and separate from their parents, they may go through periods of struggle against adults. This is a normal part of growing up, but the struggle may be harder for a child with diabetes who has to take insulin, check glucose and urine all the time, and follow a meal plan.

There are no easy solutions. It may help to talk with the child about his concerns. Talking over his feelings about having diabetes can help to ease the tension many children feel. Talking things out may help you and other family members to understand how your child feels. It also gives family members a chance to offer their support. Sometimes your child with diabetes will benefit from talking with another adult (a teacher, school counselor, doctor, nurse, social worker, or minister).

Learning about diabetes and taking on self-care tasks may help your child to come to terms with having diabetes. Often when children are diagnosed with diabetes very young, they never learn basic information about the disease. Understanding how the disease works and why they need to take insulin, check their blood glucose, and so on can help children to accept having diabetes. As your child grows and develops, both you and he will need continuing education about diabetes.

Diabetes and your child's friends

When children start school, their relationships with their friends become very important to them. Your child's attitude about diabetes can influence his friends' attitudes. If your child accepts diabetes positively, it's likely that his friends will do the same. You can help your child to develop a positive attitude by demonstrating your love, support, and understanding.

Your child's friends may be fearful because they lack information about diabetes. Encourage your child to be open about the disease with his friends. However, a child's willingness to be open about diabetes will depend on his personality. Sometimes a child with diabetes feels sensitive about being different from his friends because he has to take insulin, test blood glucose, and follow a meal plan.

Some children have checked their blood glucose or given themselves an insulin injection for show-and-tell. Older children have presented science projects on diabetes and its care. However, a child who is sensitive or shy about having diabetes may not wish to draw attention to himself in this way. Understanding your child's personality will help you to handle these situations in the way that works best for him.

Communicating with your child's school and teachers

Your child's teachers, the school nurse, and the principal of your child's school all need to know about his diabetes.

When your child starts school, changes schools, or has a new teacher, it's a good idea for parents to ask for a conference-type meeting with all of these people. This way, everyone hears the same information at the same time and their questions can be answered. Having a written plan that includes important phone numbers is also helpful.

You can get brochures for school staff from your local affiliate of the American Diabetes Association. These brochures explain diabetes and treatments for low and high blood glucose. This kind of information will help school staff to feel more secure when dealing with your child.

Ask the school staff to inform you whenever there is a change to the school schedule that affects your child's meal times or exercise routine, so you can plan ahead.

Schools' legal responsibilities regarding children with diabetes

The level of health-care assistance available at your child's school will vary. Few schools today employ a full-time school nurse. Often one school nurse covers an entire school district and in some states the role of the school nurse may no longer exist. Schools often rely on the school secretary or a health aide to provide emergency health care. Many schools have inadequate policies regarding health care for students.

Under federal law, diabetes is considered a disability, and it is illegal for schools to discriminate in any way against a person with a disability. Federal law also requires that anyone with a disability have full access to public programs, which includes the public schools. In addition, federal law entitles children with diabetes to special education services if they need them.

Federal laws that protect children with diabetes include the Rehabilitation Act of 1973, the Education for All Handicapped Children Act of 1975, and the Americans With Disabilities Act of 1992.

When a school is notified that a child has diabetes, it must do an evaluation of the child's special needs. This might require obtaining medical information from the child's doctor or health-care team. The school must prepare a plan that outlines how the child's special health-care needs will be met so that he has an equal opportunity to take part in all school programs.

The school must consult you, the child's parent, about the plan, and it cannot alter the plan without your consent. A school staff member must be designated to be responsible for implementing the plan, and other school staff must know what the plan requires them to do. The plan should be updated every year.

What if my child has low blood glucose at school?

Your child's teachers and other school staff, such as the secretary, health aide, or school nurse (if there is one) need to know the signs of low blood glucose (see *Hypoglycemia*, pages 7 and 64–65). Subtle signs can be missed unless the school staff is well informed. For example, these behaviors may be signs of undetected low blood glucose:

◆ midmorning sleepiness
◆ lack of attention in class just before lunch or in midafternoon
◆ complaints of a headache after gym

Most elementary school teachers can treat the child in the classroom by giving him a glucose tablet and crackers to eat (if the child is not treating the episode on his own).

It's a good idea to give a supply of sugar cubes, glucose tablets, crackers, or small juice boxes to your child's teacher, as well as to your child, for emergencies. You may want the gym teacher to have a supply as well.

Some teachers may send the child to the nurse, the health aide, or the principal for treatment and a blood glucose test. Find out which school staff member is responsible for helping your child to do a blood test, and ask him or her to record the test result. This will help you to monitor patterns in your child's glucose levels.

Your child's teachers should also know how to give a glucagon injection. However, many school districts do not allow school personnel to give glucagon injections. Find out what your school district's policy is when you meet with your school's staff.

When talking with the staff of your child's school, be sure to stress that your child should not be sent to the nurse's office alone. A friend should go along in case low blood glucose causes your child to become dizzy or confused.

Some children may feel anxious about low blood glucose and ask to leave the classroom a lot. They may not have learned to tell the difference between feeling anxious and having a "low." Alternatively, they may be seeking attention or trying to get out of class.

The fastest way to stop this behavior is to ask for a blood glucose test whenever the child wishes to leave the room. If blood glucose isn't low, the child should stay in class.

Handling snacks at school

Your child may need to eat one or more snacks during the school day. You may decide to send a supply of snacks to be kept at the school or to pack snacks daily with the child's lunch.

Usually your child should also eat a snack before gym class. If gym is right after a meal, the snack should be eaten after the class rather than before. Crackers with peanut butter or cheese, pretzels, apples, or small cans of juice are ideal snacks.

Some teachers have used classroom snack time to teach children about healthy eating. Instead of cookies and milk, they may serve popcorn or a cereal mix. This not only helps the child with diabetes to feel like "one of the crowd," but it also teaches healthy eating habits to the other children.

What if my child has high blood glucose at school?

It's important to explain to the staff of your child's school what the signs of high blood glucose are. (See *Hyperglycemia*, pages

> John had just started middle school and learned that lunch was served at 10:15 a.m. Because he took his insulin at 8 a.m., 10:15 was early to be having lunch. John wanted to eat lunch with his classmates, but he worried that he might have low blood glucose in the afternoon because his next scheduled snack wasn't until 3 p.m. He solved the problem by adding a small snack at 1 p.m., which he ate on his way to math class. The extra snack prevented him from having low blood glucose in the afternoon. This solution enabled John to eat with his friends and be "one of the gang."

5–6.) It may be helpful to also explain that when your child's blood glucose is running a bit high, he may need to make extra trips to the bathroom or the water fountain.

You may want to ask your child's teacher or the school nurse to tell you when your child has signs of high blood glucose. These signs may indicate that your child's insulin dosage needs to be adjusted.

Checking blood glucose at school

It used to be that if a child's diabetes was well controlled, blood glucose testing during school hours was not considered essential. But because the Diabetes Control and Complications Trial showed the importance of maintaining good glucose control, many doctors recommend that children test before lunch when they are at school. (See *New Thinking About Treating Children With Diabetes*, page 9.) Testing before taking part in a strenuous sport like basketball or football can also be useful.

Your child may feel uncomfortable about doing blood tests at school, or it may really disrupt his school routine to have to do the tests. If this is the case, ask your diabetes educator for advice about how often testing is necessary and how to fit it in during a busy school day.

School lunches and parties

Many schools make lunch menus available ahead of time, giving you and your child a chance to plan (see *How Can I Help My Child to Accept Meal Planning?* page 54).

When you talk with the staff at your child's school, you may want to mention that your child tries to avoid eating fatty foods and sweets. This will help them to be sensitive to your child's needs at snacks or parties. But teachers and other school staff should not be expected to keep an eye on what your child eats every day.

School parties can be hard on children with diabetes. Your child will want to eat the same party food that the other children are eating. Ask the teacher to let you know when a party is planned and suggest that he or she also speak to the parents of the child who is having the party. Some teachers will encourage all parents to bring party foods that all the children can eat. If

The cafeteria staff at 10-year-old Drew's school knew about his diabetes and wanted to be helpful. Every day when Drew bought his lunch, a cafeteria aide would check his tray to make sure his lunch was healthy. Drew, embarrassed by this, stopped eating his lunch. As a result, he started having low blood glucose in the early afternoon. When Drew's mother found out what was happening, she arranged to meet with the school staff and asked the cafeteria aides not to check on Drew's food choices. Drew was then able to eat his lunch without embarrassment.

you have time and know ahead what's happening in school, you might send in a bag of air-popped popcorn or pretzels so the children have some low-fat options during the party. (For more on this subject, see *Parties and Holidays*, page 56.)

Will my child have to miss a lot of school?

Your child with diabetes should not have to miss school more than other children. Frequent absences from school may be a signal that your child's diabetes is not being controlled as well as it could be.

Frequent absences may also be a sign that your child has an emotional problem. Sometimes a child may try to use diabetes as an excuse to avoid going to school. If this happens, you may want to seek advice from a doctor, social worker, school counselor, psychologist, or psychiatrist. (See *Asking for Help*, page 109.)

SHOULD I SEND MY CHILD TO DIABETES CAMP?

Going to camp can be a good experience for any child. Camps geared to children with diabetes make sure that the experience is safe and healthy. Most diabetes camps have these goals:

- ◆ giving children the opportunity to meet other children who have diabetes
- ◆ helping children to be more independent by teaching them about diabetes and about self-care

Each diabetes camp has its own way of teaching children about diabetes. Some camps use schoolroom-type lectures. Others have a much more informal structure.

Going to camp seems to help most children with diabetes. They learn more about their condition and often learn to give their own insulin injections for the first time. At camp, children with diabetes meet many other children who share the same problems. After leaving camp, children often become pen pals and continue to share their feelings and fears.

Camp can provide an opportunity for children to learn independence and assume self-care tasks. Parents can feel comfortable knowing that the camp staff is trained to handle problems related to diabetes.

For a complete list of camps for children with diabetes, contact your local affiliate of the American Diabetes Association (in the white pages of the phone book). The American Diabetes Association can also give you information about weekend trips for teens, family camps, and year-round activities.

DIABETES AND YOUR CHILD'S HEIGHT AND WEIGHT

Children, especially teenagers, are often very concerned about their appearance and may want to know how diabetes can affect it. Children with diabetes need not look any different from other children.

However, if diabetes is not well cared for, it may affect a child's height and weight. Thyroid disease may also cause growth problems (see *Thyroid Disease*, page 75). Your child's doctor should monitor his height and weight carefully.

Sudden weight loss can be a sign of uncontrolled diabetes. When the body isn't making enough insulin, it breaks down fat to obtain energy and passes more water than usual, causing weight to drop. Once your child's blood glucose levels are brought under control, he should regain the lost weight.

My child wants to lose weight

Losing weight can be hard for a plump child or teen with diabetes because he must eat regularly to cover insulin. A child with diabetes cannot go on a crash diet.

Sometimes teenagers with diabetes decide that losing weight is more important than controlling blood glucose levels. If a teen skips meals or cuts calories without reducing insulin, he can end up with severe low blood glucose. Teens may also try to lose weight by cutting down on insulin, which can cause severe high blood glucose.

If a youngster with diabetes wants to lose weight, it is best to get help from a doctor or a dietitian. Weight loss through a low-calorie diet that limits fat intake, provides the right nutrients, and controls blood glucose levels may take longer, but it will be safer.

When a lower-calorie diet is recommended, it's important to reduce insulin. Getting more exercise can also be a helpful weight-loss strategy.

Fad diets and diet pills are very popular, especially among teenage girls. However, fad diets can be harmful because they may not provide enough nutrients. In people with diabetes, a fad diet can upset blood glucose control.

Over-the-counter diet pills may work for a short time but many people soon regain weight. Because diet pills can cause dizziness, nervousness, anxiety, sleeplessness, and other side effects, they are generally not recommended for children and teens.

Joining a weight-loss program can be helpful. Teens, especially, seem to do better at weight loss in a group with other teens.

BROTHERS AND SISTERS

Siblings can be a great asset to a child with diabetes. Because brothers and sisters usually know each other well and notice unusual behavior, a sibling may be the first to pick up signs of low blood glucose.

How will having a child with diabetes affect my other children?

Because a youngster with diabetes gets a lot of attention, brothers and sisters may sometimes feel anxious or neglected. Seeing their brother or sister with low blood glucose can be frightening, especially for younger siblings, who may fear that the child with diabetes will die. Brothers and sisters may think that their angry feelings or bad thoughts caused their sibling to get sick.

It is important to talk these fears over with children and reassure them that they did not cause their sibling's diabetes. Once they are about 5 or 6, children can take part in educational sessions about diabetes and can be encouraged to help with the care of the child with diabetes.

Brothers and sisters may be afraid of getting diabetes themselves. The chance that this will happen is very slight. Studies show that about 5 out of every 100 siblings of a child with diabetes may get diabetes by age 30.

A teenager with diabetes was having a hard time accepting her insulin injections. Every morning she created a scene by refusing her insulin. The whole family's attention was on her as her 3-year-old brother watched. No one realized how this affected the younger brother until one morning he cried for his mother to give *him* an injection.

How brothers and sisters can help

Brothers and sisters can be taught the signs and symptoms of low blood glucose and can help parents watch for these signs in the child with diabetes. For example, a sibling who shares a bedroom with the child with diabetes can be taught to alert parents when the child has nightmares or sleeps restlessly. Siblings who are mature enough can help with blood and urine testing or with giving insulin injections.

But brothers and sisters are not substitute parents. Although they may be very willing to help when their sibling with diabetes needs them, they should not be forced to assume the burden of caring for their sibling.

Ten-year-old Matt, who has diabetes, was on the same soccer team as his brother Peter, 12. If Matt experienced low blood glucose during an active game, the coach always asked Peter to sit out of the game while Matt treated himself. This made Peter angry. He was willing to help if his brother needed him but didn't like being forced to sit out of the game because of Matt. When he told his father what was happening, his father asked the coach not to make Peter leave the game to help Matt.

Fourteen-year-old Anne and her 11-year-old sister Wendy played on a softball team together. One day during a game Anne noticed that Wendy was stumbling a lot and throwing the ball poorly. She gave the younger child sugar cubes and crackers. Wendy went on to hit a winning home run.

Planning meals for the family

It's a good idea for the whole family to eat the same meals instead of serving a separate meal for the child with diabetes. This helps the child with diabetes to feel part of the family. Other family members benefit by learning healthy eating habits. When siblings understand the dietary needs of the child with diabetes, they can help him to select healthy foods.

Some parents may feel that they are punishing their other children by not having sweets in the house. They buy foods for the other children that the child with diabetes can't eat. This is very hard on the child with diabetes, who may not have enough self-control to refuse to eat candy or other treats. As one teenage girl remarked, "When ice cream is sitting there, it's hard to not want it."

All children need to know that following a healthy diet is not punishment but a habit that will help them to stay well and prevent overweight and cavities. The meal plan for your child with diabetes can be flexible enough to include occasional sweet

Nine-year-old Keisha saw her two teenage brothers eating cookies and potato chips every day—foods that Keisha wasn't allowed to eat because she had diabetes. But when her parents weren't watching, Keisha would help herself to the cookies and chips. When her mother found out, she became upset with Keisha. Keisha told her mother how sad she felt when she saw the boys eating snacks that she wasn't allowed to have. A family meeting was arranged, and Keisha told her brothers how she felt. The boys agreed to cut down on eating snacks at home. Mother and Keisha talked to the diabetes educator about adjusting Keisha's insulin and meal plan so that she could have occasional desserts and treats with her brothers.

treats. Parents may also suggest to their other children that, while it's okay for them to eat sweets sometimes when they are out with their friends, they should not eat them at home.

THE TEEN WITH DIABETES

The teen years are often a challenging time for both youngsters and parents. As youngsters move toward adulthood they go through many physical and emotional changes. Children's increasing maturity and desire for greater independence can affect their diabetes care and strain relationships with their parents.

Teens and diabetes care

For the teenager with diabetes, having to take insulin, test blood glucose regularly, and stick to a meal plan can all compound the normal difficulties of puberty. It's tempting for many teens to ease up on diabetes care and try to act "like everyone else."

The teenage years are a period of developing a new identity. Many teens try to distance themselves from their families. Teens with diabetes may try to show their independence by

♦ refusing to do blood tests
♦ making up false test results
♦ bingeing on sweets or fatty foods like french fries and potato chips

Parents are often shocked, baffled, and worried by this behavior. However, with patience and a willingness to listen to the teen's concerns, parents can often help him to mature while maintaining acceptable levels of diabetes care.

Sixteen-year-old Bob had a very busy schedule with school and sports and really couldn't do more than two blood tests a day. His mother scolded him for not doing more tests, and when he went for his diabetes checkups the doctor scolded him, too. But at his most recent checkup he saw the diabetes educator, who said it was terrific that he did two blood tests a day. She didn't get upset or scold him. When she asked if Bob could try to do three tests on days when he played basketball, Bob thought he could handle that. Although Bob's care was still far from perfect, he had taken a step in the right direction.

If a teen and his parents are having a lot of problems related to diabetes care, an adult from outside the family (a coach, teacher, or nurse) may be able to provide the support the teen needs to manage his own care.

Setting realistic goals is important. If a teenager is only doing one blood test a day, negotiating with him to do two—and praising him when he does it—will be more successful than demanding he do four.

Encouraging independence

To help the teen with diabetes become independent, it is important to allow him to make decisions about his own care. Ideally, teens should already be making choices about meals and types and amounts of food.

Let go gradually and allow the teen to take responsibility, as he feels ready, for urine and blood testing and insulin injections. The teen will make mistakes but will learn from them. You can help by making sure that proper supplies and foods are available.

Show that you are still interested and concerned about your teen by asking: "How are your tests running these days?" This shows that you expect the teen to be taking care of himself, but that you want to remain involved in his care.

Encourage the teen to develop a separate relationship with the doctor, dietitian, or diabetes educator. This can help him to find a treatment plan that he can live with. You can, of course, still talk to the doctor about concerns that you may have, but suggest that your teenager go to see the health-care provider on his own.

Try to be as loving, supportive, and patient as possible. It won't be easy, but many parents whose children don't have diabetes face similar problems. Most teens weather these stormy years quite well and become successful, self-assured adults. When the changes of the teenage years are creating great distress, psychological counseling may be helpful for teens and families. (See *Asking for Help*, page 109.)

Diabetes and alcohol

Teenagers often want to try new and different things. Experimenting with alcohol is very common, even though it is illegal for teenagers to drink.

Alcohol poses special risks for people with diabetes. Drinking too much alcohol can lower blood glucose. Combining alcohol with a sugary mixer or with too much food can raise blood glucose.

Alcohol can cloud judgment. A teen who has been drinking may forget his care plan or neglect to treat low blood glucose. He may think that alcohol is making him feel "strange" when the feeling may be partly caused by plummeting blood glucose. Other

Guidelines for Alcohol Use by People With Diabetes

These guidelines are followed by many adults with diabetes who drink moderately.

◆ Know the harmful effects of alcohol. It's safest not to drink.
◆ Always carry your medical ID.
◆ If you can, make your own drink. That way, you'll know how much alcohol is in it.
◆ Have no more than two drinks.
◆ Make sure that at least one person with you knows that you have diabetes and knows the signs of low blood glucose.
◆ Check your blood glucose from time to time. This is particularly important if you are doing anything physically active like dancing, playing ball, or swimming.
◆ Drink slowly. Sometimes one drink can satisfy a craving and allow you to feel part of the crowd.
◆ The less alcohol in a drink, the better. Know the alcohol content of various kinds of liquor. Light wines often have low alcohol contents. Dry wines often have less sugar than sweeter ones. Alcohol can be diluted by mixing it with diet soda or club soda.
◆ Alcohol has no nutritional benefits. For practical purposes, however, it is usually counted as a fat (1 oz. alcohol = 1 Fat Exchange).
◆ Alcohol may make you hungry, and you may forget the importance of sticking to your meal plan. When drinking, try to avoid bingeing on party snacks and desserts.
◆ If you have a mixed drink, avoid sugar-sweetened mixers. Use club soda, water, or diet beverages.
◆ Alcohol is safest when consumed as a part of a meal or scheduled snack. Don't substitute alcohol for meals or snacks and don't drink on an empty stomach. If your meal is delayed, or you drink too much alcohol, you may have a "low."
◆ Drinking and driving may be especially dangerous for people with diabetes. This is because alcohol may increase your risk of getting low blood glucose.
◆ If you are taking any medications (such as antihistamines or cold remedies) talk to your doctor about what effect they may have on alcohol or on your diabetes control.

people may not notice the signs of low blood glucose if they think, "He's just drunk."

If a teen, knowing the risks, decides to drink alcohol, he should be aware of the guidelines in the chart on page 99.

Diabetes and tobacco use

Using tobacco in any form increases health risks. Smoking is linked to about 106,000 lung cancer deaths and about 225,000 deaths from heart disease every year. Smoking can also cause high blood pressure, allergies, and ear and sinus infections.

People with diabetes already have a higher than average risk of getting heart disease, high blood pressure, and kidney disease. Combining smoking with diabetes further increases an individual's chances of having health problems.

Some teens chew tobacco or use snuff, thinking that these habits are less hazardous to health than smoking. In fact, the body absorbs more nicotine when tobacco is chewed or inhaled than when it is smoked. Chewing tobacco and snuff can make the nose and eyes run, cause irritation of the membranes in the nose and mouth, and lead to cancer of the nose and mouth.

In spite of these health risks, however, many teens choose to smoke or chew tobacco. Parents can help teens to decide against smoking by making the facts available—and by not smoking themselves.

When a person with diabetes tries to cut down on smoking or quit, he may experience symptoms of nicotine withdrawal (drowsiness, restless sleep, irritability, headache, and hunger) that are similar to symptoms of low blood glucose.

Doctors can prescribe nicotine patches to reduce the side effects of nicotine withdrawal. Smoking cessation classes offered by high schools or community hospitals can be a source of support for those who are trying to give up tobacco use.

Diabetes and illegal drugs

Some teens are attracted to illegal drugs like marijuana and cocaine. They may believe that these drugs are safe and that drug use is fun or a sign of maturity.

Before teens with diabetes consider using illegal drugs, they should know not only their general risks but also the special risks drugs pose to people with diabetes. Like alcohol, drugs can play havoc with blood glucose levels. In some cases drugs lower glucose levels and in other cases raise them. A person's response to a drug may mask the warning signs of low blood glucose.

Marijuana can make people very hungry. Eating too much can, of course, cause overweight. The teen with diabetes also risks high blood glucose.

It may be hard for parents to get this information across without sounding "preachy." One approach may be to provide booklets about drug use that are written especially for teenagers and that suggest resources teenagers can turn to for help or additional information.

Try to have a calm discussion about drugs and listen to your child. You might tell the teen that you understand his curiosity about drugs and the pressure he may be under to try them. If your child chooses to try drugs in spite of these efforts, you may want to urge him to take precautions such as setting limits in advance, asking a friend to look for signs of low blood glucose, and checking blood glucose while using drugs.

Driving

Getting a driver's license is a big day in every teen's life. Driving should not be a problem for the teen with diabetes, but he will need a doctor's clearance and should always be prepared for low blood glucose when driving.

Glucose gels, sugar cubes, and packaged crackers should always be kept in the glove compartment. You never know when a traffic jam could delay a meal or snack!

It's a good idea to always test blood glucose before driving. If the teen feels a low blood glucose episode coming on while driving, he should park the car right away, treat the "low," and wait until he feels 100 percent.

Driving may be a problem for a person with diabetes who does not feel early warning signs of low blood glucose. Blood glucose testing before driving is essential for anyone who has this problem. Wearing an ID tag is important in case of an accident (see *Should My Child Wear a Medical ID Tag?* page 68.)

Dating

Diabetes need not prevent a teen from having a full and fun-filled social life. For many teens this will include dating.

The teen may wish to tell his date about diabetes. A brief explanation in advance may help the teen to avoid sweets at a party or clear the way for having a needed snack while out on a date. Explaining the signs of low blood glucose can help to prevent misunderstanding if the teen becomes irritable, pale, or restless.

Snacks should not be a problem on a date or at a party as long as they are included in the meal plan. The teen can ask what food is being served at a party or discuss a restaurant's menu with his date beforehand. This allows time to adjust the meal plan. Many teens bring their own sugar-free soft drinks to parties and volunteer to contribute cut, fresh vegetables to the snack table.

Eating disorders

Eating disorders most often affect teenage girls and young women. A girl who is preoccupied with her weight or who feels she has no control over her life may be more likely to get an eating disorder. Teenagers with diabetes may be at risk for eating disorders because they need to follow a meal plan and, like many teenagers, they may be concerned about gaining weight.

The two most common eating disorders in teenage girls and young women are:

- ◆ **Anorexia nervosa**. People with this disorder lose weight by starving themselves.
- ◆ **Bulimia**. People with this disorder sometimes starve themselves and sometimes go on food binges. After bingeing, they may make themselves throw up or take laxatives or water pills to get rid of all the food.

A teenager who displays several of the following signs may have an eating disorder:

- ◆ extreme thinness
- ◆ wearing of multiple layers of clothing to cover what is perceived as fat
- ◆ cracks or redness in the corners of the mouth
- ◆ dark marks on the teeth, which indicate erosion of the tooth enamel

- a callous on the third knuckle, which may be caused by using the finger to induce vomiting
- trips to the bathroom after meals or snacks
- preoccupation with food or exercise
- weight loss or decreased insulin dose without an explanation

Eating disorders can be life-threatening. If you suspect that your teenager is developing an eating disorder, notify your doctor right away.

Puberty and sexual development

Puberty produces many physical and hormonal changes as your child's body becomes that of an adult. Boys' bodies begin producing testosterone (the male sex hormone), which causes muscle development, growth of facial and body hair, and deepening of the voice. In girls, estrogen (the female sex hormone) causes menstruation and the growth of breasts and pubic hair.

These physical changes may be accompanied by emotional changes such as moodiness and irritability. Teens also usually begin to develop an interest in the opposite sex.

All children and teens grow and develop at different rates. Girls usually begin puberty at a younger age than boys. Menstrual periods typically begin at age 12 to 13. However, heredity has a lot of influence on when your child reaches puberty. At 13 or 14, many boys are still boys while others are already becoming men.

Your son's growth and development will probably be similar to his father's and your daughter's will probably be similar to her mother's. For example, if Dad's voice changed at 15, Johnny's voice will probably change at around the same age. If Mom started having menstrual periods at 11, the chances are that Suzie will also start at that age.

If diabetes is well controlled it will not affect your child's growth and development. However, your doctor should carefully monitor your child's height, weight, and physical development.

Teens with diabetes, like other teenagers, may be sexually active. They need to be informed about how to protect themselves from pregnancy and sexually transmitted diseases such as HIV infection, syphilis, and other diseases. In many communities, this kind of information is available at family planning clinics, where services are both free and confidential. Your health-care provider can help you to find a family planning clinic in your area.

Impotence (the inability to have an erection) can occur in men who have had diabetes for many years. It is extremely rare among teenage boys with diabetes, but fear of it may be present at an early age. Nerve damage caused by poor glucose control is one of the reasons men with diabetes become impotent. If your teenage son has concerns about this problem, a discussion with his doctor may help.

Career choices

Many teenagers wonder, "Will diabetes limit my career choices?" The most honest answer to this question is "yes and no." By law, a person with insulin-dependent diabetes cannot enlist in the military or pilot a commercial aircraft. With these exceptions, however, most occupations are open to people with diabetes.

Some laws excluding people with diabetes from certain types of work have been successfully challenged. For example, at one time people with diabetes could not drive commercial vehicles such as trucks or buses. Now, however, people with diabetes may be accepted as truck or bus drivers on a case-by-case basis.

Advances in the treatment of diabetes have opened professional doors. People with diabetes can now be found working in many careers, including police work and fire fighting. Like other young people, teens with diabetes should choose careers based on their talents, interests, and qualifications.

People with diabetes are protected against job discrimination by the Federal Rehabilitation Act of 1973 and by many state laws. A person who feels that he has been discriminated against may contact the American Diabetes Association for further information about these laws.

The American Diabetes Association believes that "any person with diabetes, whether insulin-dependent or non-insulin-dependent, should be eligible for any employment for which he or she is otherwise qualified."

People with diabetes are found among the leading doctors, scientists, political leaders, teachers, and lawyers in the United

States. Celebrities and sports figures who have succeeded in spite of having diabetes include:

♦ actresses Mary Tyler Moore and Jean Smart
♦ professional football players Jonathan Hayes and Wade Wilson
♦ professional basketball player Chris Dudley
♦ rock musician Bret Michaels

Marriage

Teenagers with diabetes may have concerns about marriage. Many people with diabetes are very happily married. However, the issues related to diabetes should be discussed with the prospective partner before the wedding takes place.

The partner of a person with diabetes may face some lifestyle changes. He or she must understand the need to take insulin, to stick to a meal plan, and to check blood glucose levels frequently. The partner may have to deal with mood swings that can occur with changes in blood glucose levels. Some partners may feel anxious about treating low blood glucose episodes. In many cases, partners can benefit from attending diabetes education classes.

Pregnancy

Diabetes need not prevent most women from having a family. Pregnancy does pose extra risks to both the woman with diabetes and her baby, but with good medical care women with diabetes give birth to healthy infants.

Achieving good diabetes control *before* becoming pregnant is extremely important. Uncontrolled diabetes during the first few weeks of pregnancy can cause birth defects. Prenatal care and tight control of blood glucose levels during pregnancy help to assure the birth of a healthy baby.

Teenagers may wonder whether their children will also get diabetes. As discussed in *What Is Diabetes*, research shows that some people inherit a higher risk of getting diabetes. Recent studies show that, of 100 children born to a parent with insulin-dependent diabetes, between 1 and 8 may get diabetes. A couple in which one partner has diabetes may wish to get genetic counseling before starting a family.

BUDGETING

Caring for a child with diabetes on a limited budget is a challenge, but it can be done. Your dietitian can give you some useful hints about how to prepare inexpensive, healthful meals for your entire family. As with food, when shopping for diabetes supplies, it helps to compare prices, use coupons, and buy in bulk.

One money-saving habit is reusing syringes. If you are careful and observe certain precautions, syringes for injecting insulin can be reused (see *Reusing Disposable Syringes*, page 29).

Always compare prices of supplies before buying. Companies that offer mail order diabetes supplies will vary in price, selection, and service. It pays to shop around. Four times a year, *Diabetes Forecast*, the monthly magazine of the American Diabetes Association, carries ads for companies that offer diabetes supplies in bulk by mail. The *Buyers Guide to Diabetes Supplies*, published every October in *Diabetes Forecast*, is a very useful source of information about your choices of diabetes supplies.

TRAVELING

Vacations and trips are special times. A trip means a break from school, work, and the everyday routine. Unfortunately, it doesn't mean a break from diabetes care. Diabetes never takes a vacation. The charts on pages 108 and 109 provide some useful tips that will help you to plan a safe and enjoyable trip or vacation with a child with diabetes.

COPING WITH DIABETES

Having a child with diabetes can at times be very stressful for you and your family. It can be hard at first to accept that your child has a disease that isn't going to go away and that needs care and attention every day. Caring for a child with diabetes alters your family routine and can affect relationships among family members.

Having diabetes is stressful for your child, too. Young children may think that diabetes is a punishment for something they did. It's important to try to reassure your child that having diabetes isn't her fault.

Tips For Traveling—Part I

Before you go

- If your child is taking a long trip, it's a good idea for her to have a complete medical check-up before leaving. Take a record of the check-up along on the trip. Important information in the record should include insulin dose and blood- and urine-test results.
- When making flight reservations, check the times that meals and snacks will be served. Airlines have special meals (low fat, low sugar) for people with diabetes. You may want to ask for these when you make your reservations. It's a good idea to bring extra food like crackers or fruit in case your meals are delayed or do not appear.
- If you are traveling to a different time zone, get advice from your health-care provider about how to adjust the timing of meals, insulin injections, and so on.

Packing

- Pack diabetes supplies so they are always within easy reach. Your travel kit should include fast-acting glucose tablets, regular soda, crackers, and extra syringes with alcohol wipes. Add glucagon to the travel kit on long trips.
- Insulin need not be packed in a thermos or ice chest. But insulin bottles should be kept in a cool, dry place and protected from breakage. Insulin should not be exposed to extreme heat or cold, so don't pack it in the trunk of a hot car or keep it in the glove compartment.
- An emergency kit for hypoglycemia (low blood glucose) should always be readily available when traveling. In the emergency kit should be:
  - a fast-acting sugar (such as fruit juice, sugar cubes, or glucose tablets)
  - a long-acting carbohydrate and protein (such as peanut butter or cheese crackers)
  - a glucagon kit.
- When traveling by plane, take syringes and insulin in a carry-on bag. This protects you in case your luggage is lost.
- Pack extra food, syringes, and insulin in case of travel delays.
- Your child should wear a medical ID tag, and you should carry a medical information card (see *Should My Child Wear a Medical ID Tag?* page 68).
- If you're traveling to a country where trafficking in illegal drugs is a concern, you may want to carry a letter from your child's doctor and your child's prescriptions for insulin and syringes.

Tips For Traveling—Part II

Testing on the road
The excitement of traveling, as well as the change in food and activities, may cause your child's blood glucose to run higher or lower than normal. Frequent blood testing can help you decide how to adjust insulin dosages. Doing blood and urine testing on the road shouldn't be too difficult because the equipment is portable. Many people find that testing on the road gives them peace of mind.

Dealing with emergencies
If you are traveling to a foreign country where most people don't speak English, it is helpful to learn some key phrases in the local language:
♦ "My child has diabetes." or "I have diabetes."
♦ "The child needs (I need) food/juice/sugar,"
♦ "Please call a doctor."
Your child's doctor may be able to give you the name of an English-speaking doctor or hospital in the country you are visiting. In an emergency, the American Embassy may be able to help.

Feeling loved by the whole family can help your child to accept having diabetes. Involving everyone in the family in your child's care can help to make diabetes a normal part of family life.

Parents often worry about disciplining a child with diabetes because it can be hard to tell the difference between normal misbehavior and signs of low blood glucose. It's important, however, not to treat your child with diabetes differently from your other children. Ordinary discipline should not have any effect on your child's blood glucose levels.

ASKING FOR HELP
Every family will go through times when it's hard to cope. During these difficult periods you and your family may benefit from the help of a professional counselor.

Professional counselors are trained to help people with special problems and concerns. Many people are ashamed to ask for this kind of help. Some think that asking for help makes them a failure. Others fear being labeled mentally ill.

These concerns are understandable but untrue. There is no shame in asking for help to cope with a very hard job that gives you no time off. Caring for a child with diabetes is exactly such a job. Knowing when you need extra help is a sign of mental health, not mental illness.

Counseling can make a real difference in how diabetes affects you and your child. Many families find that just one session with a counselor makes a big difference.

How do you find a counselor that you like and feel comfortable with? If your child is cared for by a health-care team, the team may include a counselor (a social worker, psychologist, or psychiatrist). Your child's doctor may be able to refer you to a good counselor. Many communities have family service organizations that offer counseling.

You may want to go to a meeting of a support group affiliated with the American Diabetes Association. These groups usually meet informally. They offer a chance for your child to meet other children with diabetes and for you to meet other parents of children with diabetes. Parents can exchange experiences, problems, and solutions. Families can see that they are not alone. Other families are facing similar challenges—and surviving.

Look in your telephone book to see if there is an American Diabetes Association chapter in your area. The American Diabetes Association also has many books, pamphlets, and other publications about diabetes. (See page 119 for more information about the American Diabetes Association.)

Conclusion

Living successfully with diabetes isn't always easy, but with discipline, patience, and good medical care, it can be done. Everything about life with diabetes is a balancing act. You have to balance food, insulin, and activity to keep blood glucose levels within a target range.

Your child with diabetes depends on you for care and support. He will follow your lead. If you can feel comfortable and positive about your child's condition, he will learn to feel the same way. If you have a "can-do" attitude when faced with life's surprises, he'll take on challenges with the same outlook.

When your child is very young, you will do all of the day-to-day tasks of caring for his diabetes. As your child grows up, it's important that he gradually learns to take on these tasks for himself. But it's also important that you stay involved in your child's care even as you let your child take on more responsibility. This, too, is a balancing act.

The child who learns to live with diabetes has to do many things that other children don't have to do and make many decisions that other children don't have to make. He learns early in life the importance of being disciplined and taking responsibility for herself.

These are lessons that can prepare your child for life as an adult. No one would choose to have diabetes in order to learn these things. But learning to live with diabetes can, ultimately, be an experience that enriches your child's life.

Glossary

Adrenaline: A hormone that helps the body to deal with stress. By making the body produce more glucose, adrenaline can raise the blood glucose level. By helping the muscles to absorb more glucose, it can also lower the blood glucose level.

Antibody: A substance that the body makes to fight infection.

Autoimmune disorder: A disease in which antibodies, instead of helping the body fight infection, attack normal parts of the body itself. For example, antibodies may attack and destroy the cells that make insulin, causing diabetes.

Beta cells: Small clumps of cells in the pancreas that make insulin. In insulin-dependent diabetes, these cells are destroyed and no longer produce insulin.

Carbohydrate: A food group. The body's preferred source of energy. There are two kinds of carbohydrates: **simple sugars**, which the body processes quickly, and complex carbohydrates, which generally take more time to digest. Simple sugars cause a rapid rise in the blood glucose level. **Complex carbohydrates** tend to cause a more gradual rise in blood glucose.

Cardiovascular: Relating to the heart and blood vessels.

Cell: The basic structural unit of all animals and plants. Cells are the physical basis of all life processes.

Cell membrane: Material that surrounds each cell. The membrane keeps in substances that the cell needs and excludes harmful ones.

Diabetes educator: A health-care professional who has specialized training in the care of diabetes. A diabetes educator may be a nurse, a dietitian, a pharmacist, a social worker, a physician, or may be trained in another health-care field. A Certified Diabetes Educator (CDE) has passed a qualifying exam and has spent a specific amount of time leaching people about diabetes.

Diabetic coma: *See* **ketoacidosis.**

Dietitian: A health-care professional who has specialized training in diet and nutrition. A Registered Dietitian (RD) has passed a qualifying exam.

Endocrine glands: Organs and groups of cells in the body that produce **hormones**. The **beta cells** that make insulin are in the pancreas, which is an endocrine gland.

Endocrinologist: A physician who specializes in the treatment of diseases caused by imbalances of hormones. Diabetes is one such disease. Some endocrinologists who specialize in treating patients with diabetes call themselves **diabetologists**.

Exchange Lists: A meal planning tool for people with diabetes. Exchange Lists divide food into six categories: starch/bread, meat, vegetable, fruit, milk, and fat. Each list consists of foods that, in the stated amounts, provide the same amount of nutrition. Any food can be "exchanged" or substituted for any other food on the same list.

Fats: A food group and a source of energy for the body. Fats do not raise blood glucose very much, but some kinds of fat raise the cholesterol level in the blood.

Saturated fat: Fat that tends to raise the cholesterol level in the blood. Usually found in foods that come from animals. Butter and lard are saturated fats. Some vegetable oils, such as palm oil and coconut oil, are also saturated fats.

Monounsaturated fat: Fat that tends to lower blood cholesterol. Olive oil and canola oil are monounsaturated fats.

Polyunsaturated fat: Fat that tends to lower blood cholesterol. Found in most vegetable oils. Soybean oil, cottonseed oil, corn oil, and peanut oil are all polyunsaturated fats.

Gingivitis: Inflammation of the gums. Gingivitis can be a long-term complication of diabetes, but it can be reduced or prevented with regular dental care.

Glucagon: A hormone produced in the pancreas. Glucagon raises blood glucose levels. It is useful for treating very low blood glucose.

Glucose: A kind of sugar. Glucose is the body's main source of energy. The digestive system makes glucose by breaking down carbohydrate.

Glycemic response: The rate and amount by which a certain food raises blood glucose.

Glycosuria: Glucose in the urine.

Glycated hemoglobin: A substance in red blood cells. Also called HbA_1 or HbA_{1c}. Measuring HbA shows what the average blood glucose level has been over the past couple of months.

Hormone: A substance made by an endocrine gland that aids growth or body functioning. **Adrenaline, glucagon,** and **insulin** are hormones.

Hyperglycemia: A high level of glucose in the blood. Common symptoms include frequent urination, excessive thirst, weight loss, increased appetite, tiredness, and blurred vision. Hyperglycemia is a sign of uncontrolled diabetes. It may be treated by giving a bigger dose of insulin or by getting exercise to lower blood glucose levels. Untreated, hyperglycemia can lead to **ketoacidosis.**

Hyperlipidemia: A high level of fats in the blood.

Hypoglycemia: A low level of glucose in the blood. Common symptoms include nervousness, headache, pallor, fatigue, weakness, nightmares, hunger, irritability, sweating, personality changes, shakiness, and confusion. Hypoglycemia must be treated quickly. Untreated, it can lead to seizures and unconsciousness. Treat with sugar to raise blood glucose levels quickly.

Insulin: A hormone made in the beta cells of the pancreas. It allows the body to use glucose for energy.

Insulin-dependent diabetes: A condition in which the pancreas stops making insulin. Individuals with this condition must get daily injections of insulin to survive. Also called type I diabetes.

Islets of Langerhans: Clusters of cells in the pancreas. The islets are made of four kinds of cells. **Beta cells** are the ones that make insulin.

Juvenile-onset diabetes: Former name for **insulin-dependent diabetes** or **type I diabetes.** The term *juvenile-onset diabetes* is no longer used.

Ketoacidosis: A serious condition that is usually caused by uncontrolled diabetes. Ketones build up in the body, slowly poisoning it. Symptoms include nausea, vomiting, fruity-smelling breath, dry skin, labored breathing, and stupor. Also called **diabetic coma.** However, a person can have ketoacidosis without being in a coma.

Ketone: A waste product made by the body when it burns fat for energy.

Ketonemia: Ketones in the blood.

Ketonuria: Ketones in the urine.

Kidney: One of a pair of organs whose most important function is to remove waste products from the blood by passing them into the urine.

Lipids: Complex fats used in the body to store and transport needed minerals.

Maturity-onset diabetes: Former name for **non-insulin-dependent diabetes** or **type II diabetes**. The term maturity-onset diabetes is no longer used.

Metabolic rate: The rate at which the body performs its chemical and physical functions.

Metabolism: All of the chemical and physical changes in the body that enable it to grow and function.

Minerals: Substances needed in small amounts to build and repair body tissues and/or to control functions of the body. Calcium, iron, potassium, and magnesium are examples of minerals.

Nephropathy: Kidney disease. People who have had diabetes for many years are at risk of getting nephropathy.

Neuropathy: Disease of the nerves. Often causes loss of sensation or movement and pain or burning in the feet and legs. May also affect nerves in other parts of the body. People who have had diabetes for many years are at risk of getting neuropathy.

Non-insulin-dependent diabetes: A condition in which the pancreas does not make enough insulin or the body does not use insulin properly. Also called type II diabetes.

Nutrient: A substance in food that is needed by the body. Proteins, fats, carbohydrates, minerals, vitamins, and water are examples of nutrients.

Ophthalmologist: A medical doctor who specializes in the care and treatment of eye diseases.

Optometrist: A nonmedical specialist who is trained to examine the eyes and prescribe lenses or exercises to correct vision problems.

Polydipsia: Increased thirst. A symptom of **hyperglycemia**.

Polyphagia: Increased appetite. A symptom of **hyperglycemia**. Can also accompany hypoglycemia.

Polyuria: Increased urination. A symptom of **hyperglycemia**.

Protein: One of three major nutrients found in food. Proteins are a source of energy. They do not have much effect on blood glucose.

Psychology: Science dealing with behavior and mental processes.

Psychologist: A health-care professional who has specialized training in the treatment of problems that cause mental and emotional distress.

Retinopathy: A disease of the retina in the eye. A complication of diabetes.

Signs: Something abnormal that can be found by an observer, such as fever based on a thermometer reading.

Social worker: A person with specialized training in helping individuals and families to solve practical and emotional problems.

Symptoms: Something abnormal that a person can feel, such as abdominal pain.

Type I diabetes: *See* **Insulin-dependent diabetes.**

Type II diabetes: *See* **Non-insulin-dependent diabetes.**

Vitamins: Substances needed in small amounts for normal body growth and functioning.

The American Diabetes Association is the nation's leading voluntary health organization concerned with diabetes and its complications. The Association is working to prevent and cure diabetes; provide information to patients and their families, health professionals, and the general public; and lead advocacy efforts on behalf of people affected by diabetes. Founded in 1940, the Association has an affiliate office in every state and services in more than 800 communities across the country.

You can find information about summer camps for children with diabetes and local programs and support groups by contacting your state American Diabetes Association affiliate. Affiliates can also tell you how to find a quality diabetes education program in your area. Their number is in the white pages listing for American Diabetes Association.

The American Diabetes Association also publishes resources for people with diabetes. You can obtain a publications catalog or purchase publications by calling 1-800-232-3472. As a parent of a child with diabetes, you may be interested in these publications:

- *Grilled Cheese at Four O'Clock in the Morning* For ages 8–12, this story of a young boy who develops diabetes may help your child deal with his or her fears and frustrations of living with diabetes.
- *It's Time to Learn About Diabetes* A workbook for children interested in learning how diabetes affects their body and how to take care of themselves.
- *The Take-Charge Guide to Type I Diabetes* An "owner's manual" for young adults and adults taking care of diabetes on their own.
- *Necessary Toughness* The story of Jonathan Haye's diagnosis of diabetes and his success as a college and professional football player.
- *The Fitness Book for People With Diabetes* For all people with diabetes, this guide shows how to include a regular exercise program as part of your diabetes self-care. Contains a section on competitive and high-risk sports and profiles of young athletes.

The following books are available from other publishers and may be found in bookstores.

- *Psyching Out Diabetes* by Richard Rubin, June Biermann, and Barbara Toohey. A questions-and-answers book on handling the emotional issues of diabetes. Published by Lowell House.
- *Don't Shoot the Dog* by Karen Pryor. A guide to using positive reinforcement to shape the behavior of children, students, and other living creatures. Published by Bantam Books.

Index

The authors work together as coordinators of the diabetes program at Children's Hospital of Pittsburgh and have been friends for many years. *Raising a Child With Diabetes: A Guide for Parents* is their second book for the American Diabetes Association.

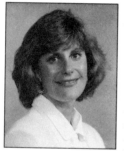

Linda M. Siminerio, RN, MS, CDE, has worked with children with diabetes for almost 25 years as a diabetes educator. She received a bachelor's degree in nursing from Pennsylvania State University and a master's degree in child development and child care from the University of Pittsburgh and is completing a doctoral degree in health education from Pennsylvania State University. Her doctoral research is in diabetes education in pediatric populations. Ms. Siminerio volunteers with the American Diabetes Association, serving on committees and as national senior vice president. She has three children.

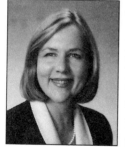

Jean Betschart, RN, MN, CDE, has been a diabetes educator since 1980. She was named Outstanding Health Professional Educator in 1994 by the American Diabetes Association. Ms. Betschart received a bachelor's degree in nursing and a master's degree as a clinical nurse specialist in parent-child nursing from the University of Pittsburgh. She is past president of the American Association of Diabetes Educators and has volunteered for the American Diabetes Association at the state and national level. Ms. Betschart developed insulin-dependent (type I) diabetes during late adolescence. She has three children.